ALLEN CARR

with

ROBIN HAYLEY

THE EASY WAY TO ENJOY EXERCISE

ALLEN CARR

with

ROBIN HAYLEY

THE EASY WAY TO ENJOY EXERCISE

Get fit without willpower

SIRIUS

SIRIUS

This edition published in 2025 by Sirius Publishing, a division of
Arcturus Publishing Limited,
26/27 Bickels Yard, 151–153 Bermondsey Street,
London SE1 3HA

ISBN: 978-1-3988-1743-2
AD010636US

Printed in the UK

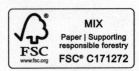

CONTENTS

DON'T SKIP THIS IMPORTANT

INTRODUCTION

BY ROBIN HAYLEY, GLOBAL CHAIRMAN & SENIOR THERAPIST, ALLEN CARR'S EASYWAY

We all want to be fit and know that exercise is essential for our physical health. But what if it feels like a chore instead of a fulfilling experience? Why is it so difficult to stay motivated and continue with an exercise plan? In this book, we explore the physical, psychological, and social aspects of exercise, and why so many people find it challenging to keep at it without calling on huge amounts of willpower. How long will our resolve last? Doesn't it frequently flag and, more often than not, disappear after a period of "being good?" Understanding the psychology of exercise will enable you to find it easy not only to become fit but also to thoroughly enjoy remaining so. No doubt you find that hard to believe, but read on and all will be explained.

We will also look at practical strategies, tips, and advice on how to overcome barriers you may have encountered previously, ensuring that exercise becomes a genuinely rewarding and sustainable part of your life. Whether you're in good shape already but not enjoying the process of keeping that way, or you need to exercise more but struggle to become motivated, this book will provide you with the insight and practical guidance you need to develop the right relationship with exercise and achieve your desired fitness and body shape without the need for willpower.

WHAT ARE OUR CREDENTIALS?

Allen Carr's reputation in the field of addiction treatment and behavioral change was built on his unparalleled success in helping smokers to quit. His Easyway method was so successful that it quickly became, and remains, a global phenomenon. From the earliest days of Easyway, Allen was inundated with requests from sufferers of numerous other addictions and problems, imploring him to help them. By the turn of the century, he had assembled a team of highly skilled and dedicated therapists who went on to help him apply his method to a variety of issues and to deliver Allen Carr's Easyway to millions of people all over the world.

We have ensured that all our books are entirely faithful to Allen Carr's original method and it's an honor for me to be writing this introduction. Rest assured, once you've read it, I'll leave you in Allen's capable hands. I consider myself extremely privileged to have worked closely with Allen on Easyway books while he was still alive, gaining insight into how the method could be applied to a growing list of issues and addictions, and together we explored and mapped out its future evolution. There is nothing in our books that Allen didn't write or wouldn't have written if he were still with us, and the updates, anecdotes, and analogies that are not his own—that were contemporized or added later—are written in Allen's voice to complement the original text and method.

We've been successfully treating behavioral issues and addictions with phenomenal success over the past 40 years. Easyway's senior team and I were inspired to join Allen's mission for one simple reason: his method transformed our lives. Like all Allen Carr's Easyway therapists across the world, we became involved with Easyway as a result of being set free from our own addictions. Allen reveled in enabling people to escape from a whole variety of addictions and problems, and many of them were so inspired that they contacted him to offer their help to spread the method. It was the ideal field from which to recruit, and it was a pleasure to work with Allen in assembling a remarkable senior therapist team that set about applying the method to as many issues as possible.

The varied background of behavioral issues and drug-taking history of our senior therapist team, far from deterring Allen from recruiting them, actually encouraged him to do so. If he was impressed by your drive, enthusiasm, ability, and accomplishments, he considered it a great bonus if you had previously experienced the misery of other issues to which Easyway could be applied. He was acutely aware that it would be extremely difficult to apply his method to the full range of behavioral issues and addictions without the direct involvement of people who had experienced them first-hand. Whether the issue was addiction to nicotine, alcohol, cocaine, cannabis, heroin, sugar, social media, or gambling; or problems with weight, eating, fear of flying, sleep, or debt, personal experience of these enabled Allen and his team to apply the method accordingly. This book is the result of that process, and I'm delighted that we now have the solution for anyone whose well-being has been undermined by an inability to enjoy exercise. How can we be so confident?

SIMPLE: THIS METHOD WORKS!

Our motivation for putting the method in writing, as well as creating our on-line video program, was to ensure that anyone, anywhere in the world, regardless of their personal circumstances, could benefit from *Allen Carr's Easy Way to Enjoy Exercise.*

Allen Carr's Easyway books have led tens of millions of people to freedom, and everything you need in order to become one of them is in front of you right now.

Many people who are unfamiliar with the method, or who have never met people who have benefited from Easyway, assume that some of the claims made about it are exaggerated. That was certainly my reaction when I first heard them. I was incredibly fortunate to have had my life saved by Allen Carr. There is no doubt that had my addictions not brought me into contact with Allen and his amazing method in the 1990s, I would have barely made it to the 21st century, let alone be here today!

I'm incredibly proud to have led the team which, over the past 25 years, has spread Allen's method all over the world. Whatever the issue, this method helps those in need in a simple, relatable, and plain-speaking way. As you're about to discover, Allen Carr's Easyway is the master of all behavioral issues. Now, without further delay, let me pass you into the safest of hands: Allen Carr and his "Easyway."

Robin Hayley M.A. (Oxon), M.B.A., M.A.A.C.T.I.
Chairman, Allen Carr's Easyway (International) Ltd

Chapter 1

THE KEY

Do you find it hard to maintain a regular exercise routine? Do you have a burning desire or desperate need to get fitter but find that your desire and desperation quickly turn to resistance, lethargy, and inertia? If only there were a way to make exercise something you look forward to as much as relaxing on the sofa. Good news! There is. And you have found it.

We all know that exercise is good for us. You don't have to be a finely tuned athlete to appreciate the benefits, and you don't have to work out vigorously every day to feel those benefits, either. Even a small amount of exercise can make a big difference to how you feel about life, as well as to your general health, mental health, and wellbeing.

Yet for some of us, our relationship with exercise is complicated. We love the idea of it and we know that it can help us feel great, but something changes when it comes to actually doing it. Whether we begin to take action and exercise more for a short period or simply fail to get going, we make excuses, find other things to do, and put it off again and again. Sound familiar?

Millions of people are going through the same tug-of-war with exercise. They want to do it. They know it will make them feel better. Yet something is holding them back. Ask them what that "something" is, and they might say it's a fear that it'll be grueling or even painful, but in most cases, it's not as severe as that. It's just a creeping lethargy that always seems to overpower the urge to exercise.

The less you exercise, the more lethargy and fatigue set in, and you suffer in three ways:

1. The lack of exercise impacts your fitness, health, body shape, and mobility.

2. That impact on your fitness, health, body shape, and mobility makes it even harder to exercise and makes you more lethargic.

3. Your inability to overcome the lethargy leaves you feeling like a weak-willed failure, which in turn, impacts your mental health and self-esteem.

All these factors result in greater susceptibility to injury, physical illness, depression, anxiety, and other issues. They create a perfect storm for all these and other negative outcomes, which leads to progressively worse lifestyle choices, behavioral issues, and even addictions.

The solution is simple in theory: overcome the lethargy and you'll receive the physical and mental benefits of exercise and escape from that guilt-ridden descent into despair. But if you found it that simple in practice, you would be doing it already, wouldn't you and you wouldn't be reading this book?

So, how can this book help you overcome lethargy, happily commit to regular exercise, and enjoy the physical and mental benefits it brings?

AN OPEN MIND

This book is the key. If you use the key correctly and follow the instructions, you will escape the mental prison you are now in, take control of your life and start to look forward to exercising as a great pleasure that improves your well-being and enables you to enjoy a longer, happier, and more fulfilled life. What's more, you won't have to use willpower or make any sacrifices. On the contrary, you will find this transformation easy, painless, and enjoyable.

The key is a method that has helped people who, like you, have found themselves caught in a vicious spiral of lethargy, inactivity, and frustration by removing the mental blocks that make exercising seem like a chore.

Reading this book will help you understand what is going on in your mind and why, enabling you to change your mindset so that you look forward to exercising with the same enthusiasm that you might look forward to engaging in your favorite pastimes.

Most important, it will make this transformation easy. You won't have to rely on willpower, which is ultimately counterproductive, nor will you have to make any sacrifices or go through any mental or physical trauma. What's more, once you've embarked on this transformation and established this new mindset, you will never be tempted to return to your previous life.

You may think that sounds too good to be true. Fitness methods are full of exaggerated claims and false promises. You probably know that from experience. The truth is that you have the power to change regardless of who you are and what your personal circumstances may be. What you need is the right mental approach. And that's what Allen Carr's Easyway is all about. Above all, you need to start with an open mind.

THE SIMPLE TRUTH

The struggle you have with exercise is remarkably similar to the struggle smokers have with nicotine and problem drinkers have with alcohol. It is riddled with contradictions. Smokers and problem drinkers wish they could quit and yet can't stand the thought of life without their drug. They believe it is the source of comfort, even though they know it is the cause of their misery. In fact, the same mental struggle applies with all addictions.

You know that exercise will make you feel healthier and happier, yet the thought of doing it is daunting. Doing anything else instead, or nothing at all, seems more appealing at the time, yet it leaves you feeling frustrated and disappointed, and it can become a dark shadow that looms in the back of your mind.

Despite these obvious contradictions, the same pattern repeats itself over and over again. Smokers know they should quit and heavy drinkers know they should at least cut down, if not quit altogether, but they fear they will feel deprived and so be forced to employ massive willpower. You know you should exercise but dread the huge effort you are convinced you'll need to make and end up in a state of inertia, incapable of doing anything about it. You know that doing nothing is a recipe for disaster and that makes you feel impotent and even more hopeless.

You have probably worked that out and yet still can't seem to overcome the lethargy. The temptation to do nothing rather than exercise is too great. It's as if you are being pinned down by a powerful monster.

This monster is ingenious. It wraps you up in confusion, twists the truth, and tricks you with convincing illusions. The purpose of this book is to help you destroy that monster and break free from the miserable, repetitive cycle of avoiding or not sustaining exercise.

It's good to relax from time to time, to let your mind and body unwind and enjoy some calm and rest. But that alone is not a formula for happiness. You need balance, a mixture of activity and inactivity, one feeding the other. Without this balance, your body and mind begin to suffer, with negative physical results compounded by negative emotions such as disappointment, frustration, self-criticism, low self-esteem, and a negative body image.

When you consider the thoroughly unpleasant consequences of perpetual inactivity, which no doubt played a part in your picking up this book, it's clearly not the pleasure of doing nothing that keeps you from exercising. Initially, you might feel relieved that you don't have to exert yourself, but as the physical and mental downsides get worse and worse, it begins to feel more like a prison you cannot escape from rather than a lifestyle choice driven by pleasure.

There is something else, like an unseen force driving you to make excuses and do nothing. A mental monster. It's the same for people with drug addictions, such as nicotine, alcohol, cocaine, heroin, sugar, or caffeine. They start out thinking they are in control, but as the addiction takes hold, they begin to realize that they don't control the drug, the drug controls them.

It's fair to assume that you do not feel in control or you wouldn't be reading this book. You have probably tried to tackle the problem already and failed. No matter how determined you were to begin with, you seemed to lack the willpower to sustain your efforts for long and this left you feeling powerless.

This book will reveal to you two very important truths:

YOU ARE <u>NOT</u> POWERLESS AND
YOU DO <u>NOT</u> LACK WILLPOWER

The reason you have struggled to overcome your problem with exercise until now is simply because you were following the wrong method.

ACKNOWLEDGE THE PROBLEM

Perhaps you have a physically demanding job and the thought of introducing an exercise routine into your day seems absurd since you collapse on the sofa whenever you have any free time. You feel like a desperate soul, lost in the desert, who has finally plunged into the shaded, watery cool of an oasis. Surely you have exercised enough to simply crash for the night? It's a good point. But how is that going for you?

As an example, let's look at the nursing profession. Nurses work long hours in a physically demanding job, so surely they should be some of the fittest members of society. Yet recent research indicates that about half of US nurses are overweight or obese. A lack of access to healthy food and easy access to unhealthy food in the workplace, combined with fatigue after those long, hard hours at work, can cause a downward spiral in health, well-being, and fitness, which in turn leads to greater fatigue and so on. Physical exertion becomes harder, mobility suffers, and so does the rate at which the nurse burns energy.

Exhausted, it's easy to see how bad food choices sneak into leisure time as well as work time.

Lest you think I am picking on nurses, I should be clear that I am merely using them as an example of how even those who physically exert themselves in the most demanding circumstances every day can still end up with a fitness problem. I should also point out that the fitness of the general population is even worse. It is estimated that more than two-thirds of US adults are overweight or obese! The UK and Ireland don't fare much better, with just under two-thirds being in the same unfortunate shape.

There is of course more to fitness than exercise alone, and I'll expand on this in due course.

YOU CANNOT "OUT-EXERCISE" A POOR DIET

Having a holistic approach to enjoying exercise is important and involves looking at what you eat, what you drink, and even how you sleep.

Nobody likes to admit they can't control their behavior. While sometimes we don't like the choices we are given, or even those that we appear to make, we like to think we at least have the freedom to choose. Problems like struggling to overcome our reluctance to exercise make us feel as though we have lost this freedom, and that can make us very self-critical. We feel ashamed; we lose self-respect; we feel confused by our apparent weakness. These are difficult feelings to live with, so we pretend they are not happening. We go into denial, bury our head in the sand, and suppress our feelings. But we can't hide from the problem.

It just doesn't go away, does it?

DENYING YOU HAVE A PROBLEM CREATES A BURDEN THAT ONLY MAKES THE PROBLEM WORSE

It can also make you feel very alone. There really is nothing shameful about not exercising, but that is not the real issue. It's debilitating wanting to achieve something but feeling unable to. And when the only thing you can see holding you back is yourself, it's natural to assume that there is something wrong with you: a weakness in your personality or perhaps even in your genetic makeup.

Trying to bury the issue just compounds it. To tackle any problem, the first essential step is to acknowledge that you have it—or that it has you. The fact that you are reading this book is a sign that you have already done that and so you are off to a flying start. Now, you just need to follow the method.

The solution is in your mind. You need to break the cycle of lethargy, inactivity, and disappointment. As you absorb the contents of this book, be honest about your feelings and be prepared to open your mind to some truths that may initially seem hard to accept.

Remember, you are not alone—far from it. Avoiding exercise, or even feeling incapable of it, is a global problem, threatening the health and happiness of billions of people. As you open your mind to the truths contained in this book, you will free yourself from this trap.

It will also become apparent that your problem is not the result of some failing in your personality or genetic makeup. That is an illusion. As I will explain, there are several factors at work that can make you believe such myths. Once you can recognize these factors, dispelling the illusions becomes easy. Most people go through life completely ignorant of these factors, so they struggle with their problems without ever becoming free. The more you allow yourself to open up and unravel the myths, the more you will understand that you can regain control and live the life you want. And you can do all this without willpower.

WHY EASYWAY WORKS

I've mentioned the similarities between aversion to exercise and addiction. Easyway is a scientifically proven method of escaping from addiction. That's why it has been recommended by the National Institute for Health and Care Excellence (NICE), which is the UK government authority that approves methods of helping people with health issues, and why Easyway is now available on the UK National Health Service (NHS) at taxpayers' expense. It is the first branded method ever to gain such approval since NICE was set up in 1999–a truly amazing statistic! It is also a partner of the World Health Organization (WHO) and global health insurers. There is no possible greater scientific endorsement and it has been achieved for one reason only:

EASYWAY WORKS

It is built on the realization that addiction hijacks your natural instincts and logical mind to create the illusion that the "fix" you turn to for relief is a genuine pleasure or comfort, whereas the truth is that it is actually the cause of your problem in the first place.

That was the revelation that gave rise to this method. I was a confirmed nicotine addict, choking my way through 60 to 100 cigarettes a day and resigned to a premature death. I was under the misapprehension that smoking was a habit I had acquired and lacked the willpower to kick. I assumed it was a problem I was stuck with. The moment of revelation came when I realized that smoking wasn't a habit, it was an addiction.

In that moment, I saw with extraordinary clarity that my inability to quit smoking was neither a weakness in my character nor some magical quality in the cigarette. It was the trap of addiction, fooling me into seeking relief in the very thing that was causing my misery.

This led to two indisputable conclusions:

- Smoking provides no genuine pleasure or comfort.

- Stopping therefore involves no sacrifice or deprivation.

I quit there and then and never felt the temptation to smoke again.

I gave the method its name "Easyway" because it requires no willpower, no substitutes, no gimmicks. It simply enables smokers to become happy non-smokers by unraveling the brainwashing that convinces them that smoking is a genuine pleasure or comfort.

The method is phenomenally successful in helping smokers to quit, with clinics in more than 50 countries and a book that has been translated into over 40 languages.

Once any addict rids themselves of the illusion that they are making a sacrifice by stopping, they find it easy to quit because they don't feel deprived, and they are happy to be free.

I realized that this method would work for all addictions and went on to apply it successfully to alcohol, weight issues, other drugs, and even "drugless" addictions like gambling and digital/technology addictions. The key is understanding that all addictions are mainly a condition of the mind. The difficulty in stopping is around 1 percent physical and 99 percent psychological.

Easyway unravels the misconceptions that drive you to do something that destroys you in the belief that it helps you or gives you pleasure. Can you see how this principle applies to your problem with exercise? At the moment, when you make your excuse to avoid it, you believe you are choosing an easier option. But almost immediately after you have made that choice, you begin to feel disappointed in yourself, frustrated by your apparent weakness, and miserable that you have let yourself down again. Of course, relaxation can be genuinely enjoyable and pleasurable, as can exercise. The key is to ensure that when you relax and rest, you are able to do so without guilt or causing yourself harm, and that is only possible once you have discovered the joy of exercise. The way to do that is to explore and exploit the qualities of relaxation, fun, and recreation that exercise offers.

WHAT THIS BOOK WILL DO FOR YOU

Unlike some fitness methods, this book is not about scaring you into action. You probably know enough about the health risks associated with a lack of exercise that you would have no problem motivating yourself if that alone were the issue. I know from experience that scare tactics don't work. In fact, they are a hindrance. You probably already feel powerless and miserable, compounding these feelings with fear and guilt would only exacerbate the problem.

This book will:

- Change the way you think about exercise.

- Show you how to overcome your aversion to it easily and painlessly.

- Open your mind to enjoy the genuine pleasures it brings.

- Enable you to take back control.

As you absorb it and develop your understanding of how the psychology works, you will begin to make sense of the feelings you have suffered in relation to your aversion to exercise and/or your inability to sustain it as an enjoyable part of your lifestyle. In particular, the confusion and mental tug of war between wanting to exercise and not wanting to will be resolved.

This is not a fitness manual. At the end of the book, you will not be physically fitter, but the key is that you will feel mentally prepared and excited to embrace exercise as a regular and enjoyable part of your life. You will also probably be empowered and inspired to examine what other areas of your life might be dramatically improved, which will make exercise even more enjoyable.

As well as not using scare tactics, I can give you several other assurances: you won't be talked down to or patronized; you won't be tricked with gimmicks; you won't feel deprived; and by the end, you won't feel you have to make any sacrifices.

There is no pain with this method. In fact, have you ever heard fitness gurus claim, "No pain, no gain?" Well, forget it. The fear of pain is a major cause of aversion to exercise. A dog doesn't feel pain when it exercises. On the contrary, it loves every minute. And so will you when you have finished reading this book.

By explaining how the mental process works and setting out simple, step-by-step instructions to help you change your mindset, this book will show you how to enjoy a healthier, happier life.

THE INSTRUCTIONS

As you go through the book, you will come across a series of instructions. If you miss one of these instructions or fail to follow any of them, you will not be using the method. If you skip ahead or read the book in a different order other than it is written, you will undermine your chances of success.

Easyway is the key to freeing yourself from the trap you are in, and it works like the combination to unlock a safe: if you don't apply all the numbers in the correct order, the lock will not open. If you do, it will. This brings us nicely to the:

FIRST INSTRUCTION:
FOLLOW ALL THE INSTRUCTIONS

Chapter 2

THE "A" WORD

IN THIS CHAPTER

•*A PROBLEM IN THE MIND* •*FALSE PLEASURES* •*WHY AVERSION TO EXERCISE IS ADDICTIVE*

When you started reading this book, you may have had a number of preconceptions. You may have heard the claim that Easyway works without willpower, substitutes or any unpleasant side effects, and thought that sounds great. You may not have expected to come across the word 'addiction' in the first chapter.

It's natural to balk at the word "addiction." The common perception of an addict is someone with serious alcohol, cocaine or heroin issues. These days, though, we have much more knowledge about the way the brain works and how it can be "remolded" through conditioning, and there is general recognition that addiction afflicts far more people than those whom society might describe as alcoholics or junkies. The human mind is highly susceptible to brainwashing, whether through drugs or other forms of conditioning, such as advertising, propaganda and peer pressure.

Perhaps you think all this talk of addiction is a bit much. What's addiction got to do with you? You just have a bit of a weakness committing to exercise, right? It's not that serious! Maybe you don't feel miserable. You just want to be able to exercise more often and feel better about doing so. So what's stopping you?

Isn't that the problem? There is something stopping you that you can neither identify nor understand. That is precisely how smokers and problem drinkers feel about their inability to quit. In fact, it's the way all addicts feel. Rather than seeing your inability to commit to exercise as a personal weakness, the key is to recognize it as an addiction to the things you do instead—the things that pull you away from exercise and make you feel less motivated.

As I will explain later, there are all sorts of addictions affecting millions of people and causing them the same problems that you are experiencing. By identifying your addictions and freeing yourself from them, you will find that your aversion to exercise disappears, and you will find it incredibly easy and enjoyable to do it. In fact, you will find it impossible to resist!

CORRECTING YOUR MINDSET

Don't worry if you're not comfortable with the word 'addiction' in this context. I use the term because it is useful in understanding what is going on in your mind. Can you acknowledge the possibility that you have developed an addiction-like tendency towards immobility, an addiction-like tendency to minimizing recreational effort, fueled perhaps by an addiction to certain foods and drinks? There is no shame in that. Don't feel bad about it. Don't we all tend to take the lift rather than the stairs, look for that parking spot closest to where we're going, use the car or bus rather than walk most of the time, or get the taxi to drop us right outside our destination, rather than hop out sooner and enjoy a brisk walk and some fresh air?

THE PROBLEM IS 1 PERCENT PHYSICAL AND 99 PERCENT MENTAL

What you choose to call the problem is not the point. What is essential is that you acknowledge that you have a problem that results in not doing enough exercise. It's nothing to feel guilty about. Millions of people have the same problem, it's just that most of them don't want to admit it.

The problem does not begin and end with an aversion to exercise. That is how the problem becomes apparent, but there are underlying factors that create that aversion. Together, we will identify those factors, bring them out in the open and give you the tools to remove them.

I'm not going to try to blind you with science, so don't worry. The following explanation is about as technical as I will get in this book. Addictions take hold when parts of the brain known as the "reward pathways" are corrupted. Reward pathways are triggered by naturally occurring hormones to make us feel good when we do something healthy or beneficial, thus encouraging us to keep doing it. When we become addicted to drugs such as nicotine, cannabis, cocaine, heroin or alcohol, we experience a feeling of dissatisfaction soon after each dose we take. This is the sensation of the drug leaving our body, otherwise known as withdrawal. When the drug is taken again, the dissatisfied feeling of withdrawal is temporarily relieved, and the reward pathways mistakenly respond as they would if we had done something that is beneficial. They do not take into account that all the drug did was temporarily relieve the discomfort the previous dose caused.

This is how the reward pathways become corrupted and how addictions establish themselves. Addictive drugs and addictive behaviors don't just corrupt the reward pathways, they bombard them, overloading them to the extent that they become dysfunctional. Eventually, the reward pathways are so numbed by this bombardment that genuine pleasures hardly register at all unless accompanied by the drug. Happiness, sadness, stress or relaxation are accompanied by an additional layer of restlessness and emptiness unless the drug is taken. Each time the drug is taken, this restlessness or emptiness is relieved and it feels like the drug has delivered a boost, so the brain is fooled into regarding it as a source of pleasure and relief. So, when you experience withdrawal from the drug again and the restless feeling returns, your brain triggers cravings for more. You take the drug again and experience another false high. It's like wearing tight shoes just for the relief you feel when taking them off.

This false high is always followed by a low, sometimes called a crash. Genuine pleasures don't do this. They give you a lasting high and don't leave you feeling low or guilty afterward.

FALSE PLEASURES

It's not just addictive drugs like nicotine, cannabis, cocaine, heroin and alcohol that have this effect on your brain. Other stimulants such as caffeine, refined sugar, and processed carbs have the same effect, as do certain behaviors such as gambling, playing computer games and compulsive shopping.

People have all sorts of addictions. Modern life is full of them, and they all trap their victims in the same way to produce symptoms that are consistent across the board: irrational irritability and evasiveness, both of which are classic traits of guilt and shame.

All addicts are burdened with guilt and shame. They might not admit it since denial is also a fundamental trait. The mental low resulting from these negative emotions is accompanied by a physical low—a restless, empty feeling as the body withdraws from its last fix. When you get your next fix, this restless feeling is partially relieved, making you think you have given yourself a genuine boost. Your brain remembers that the fix gave you a boost and is fooled into regarding the fix as a source of pleasure and relief.

The process is an ingenious assault on your mind, which twists reality and traps you in a web of illusions. And it can be caused by any of the addictive substances and behaviors that we are bombarded with every day. One of the aims of this book is to help you recognize the false pleasures that you have been bombarded with and see through the illusions that keep you going back for more.

WHY AVERSION TO EXERCISE IS ADDICTIVE

Why do you feel bad when you skip exercise? Is it because you have let yourself down? If that is the case, why not just stop letting yourself down, do the exercise and dispel the negativity. It's not that simple, is it? Why not? Nobody is holding a gun to your head. Why do you keep making choices that leave you feeling worse? Isn't it because you think you are choosing an easier, more pleasurable option?

Whenever you choose not to exercise, it is because you perceive the alternative as more appealing, even if the alternative is doing absolutely nothing. So, when you make that choice, there is a moment of relief, which feels like a momentary high. But it is soon followed by a low. This is the classic addiction cycle. Guilt and shame then follow, coupled with confusion because you can't understand why you keep making this choice. You don't actually *want* to make this choice. At the end of a lazy day, far from feeling rested, you trudge up the stairs to bed like a zombie on its last legs.

Added to this, you have denied yourself the feel-good hormones, known as endorphins, that the body releases after exercise. While drug addicts take a chemical which gives them an illusory boost, you create the same responses in your mind by avoiding something that will give you a genuine high. Drug addicts add badness while you are taking away goodness. The net effect is the same: suffering. The reasons for inflicting this misery on yourself are the same too.

AVOIDING EXERCISE DOESN'T CURE THE LOW, IT CAUSES IT

THE MORE YOU AVOID IT, THE MORE THE PHONY PLEASURE TURNS TO MISERY.

In order to resolve this issue, you need to break this vicious circle. If you don't, a problem that starts off seeming minor and under control can quickly grow to dominate your life. That dream of taking regular exercise will become more and more remote. You will feel ever more miserable, and you will feel increasingly powerless to do anything about it.

OPEN YOUR MIND

There is a widespread belief that avoiding exercise, while clearly not healthy, is not a serious threat, just as drinking alcohol, though clearly not healthy, is an accepted social norm that only causes serious problems for the unfortunate few. From childhood, we are brainwashed into thinking that alcohol has magical properties, giving you confidence, helping you unwind, making you more sociable, etc. We are "treated" to alcohol on special occasions, which makes us feel grown up. The message is clear: this stuff is special.

It's the same story with sugary foods. Cakes, sweets, biscuits and chocolate are all given to us as 'treats'. Naturally, we turn to these things for comfort. As an adult, you can indulge your needs whenever you feel like it. And the more you indulge yourself, the more you want it. Why?

BECAUSE IT'S ADDICTIVE

It's like a mosquito bite that you can't resist scratching. If you don't scratch it, the itch nags away at you and if you do, the itch gets worse. As long as you believe that the only way to stop the itch is to scratch it, you will keep scratching and the itch will keep getting worse.

So many modern-day problems, like sleep deprivation, compulsive consumption and addictions such as gambling and gaming, are caused by this same process of brainwashing, which creates a cyclical trap.

The "pleasure" you think you get is an illusion created by a subtle combination of brainwashing and the mental effects of addiction, which have physical repercussions. When you started this book, you probably didn't expect to learn about addiction. By the end of the book, you will see very clearly that an addictive process is the root cause of your problem. For now, it may still be rather confusing. That's understandable. Don't worry. I'm not suggesting for a moment that you need to stop drinking alcohol (unless you would like to), or stop eating refined sugar or processed carbs (unless you would like to)—I'm just suggesting that fine-tuning what you eat and drink, even marginally, can make a huge difference. If you understand this book and follow the instructions, Easyway will change your mindset and you will find it easy and enjoyable to achieve your goals. In order to do that, you need to keep an open mind.

SECOND INSTRUCTION: OPEN YOUR MIND

Regardless of what you may be thinking now, accept that the preconceptions you had when you started this book might be wrong. Allow your mind to open, so that it can let go of the illusions that have blocked your thinking until now and free to accept truths that may contradict your previous beliefs.

Chapter 3

IT'S ONLY NATURAL

*Different people have different reasons for wanting to
exercise. Understanding your motivations will help you
remove the factors that prevent you from doing so.*

Why do you want to exercise? We live in a world where automation
makes it easy to do nothing. You can control so many things
from the comfort of your sofa. With minimal effort, you can buy
groceries, order food, listen to music, watch TV, educate yourself,
chat with friends, control the central heating, etc.

Outside we have cars, lifts and escalators that transport
us around without having to move a muscle. Doors open
automatically, taps and hand dryers turn on by themselves. So
why the need to exercise? What is the motivation behind your
desire to make your muscles work?

That may strike you as a stupid question but the road to
unhappiness is lined with apparently stupid questions that we

never stop to ask ourselves, such as: "Do I actually like the way cannabis makes me feel?"; "Is this cigarette really making me feel relaxed?"; "Do I really want to drink more alcohol?"; and, "Am I really happier when I skip exercise and spend the evening on the sofa?"

As you absorb the contents of this book, I will ask you to ponder some basic questions. Please don't dismiss these as stupid. It's only by considering the basic issues that you develop an understanding of certain basic truths. Once you have that understanding, escaping from the trap you're currently in will be easy.

EXERCISE FOR APPEARANCE

One common reason for wanting to exercise is to look good, or perhaps a better way of putting it is to look the way you want to look. It's terribly sad that so many people are unhappy with how they look.

There is a common perception of what an attractive human body looks like. Slim, toned, youthful.... These are the general criteria for a beautiful body for people today.

That hasn't always been the case and it's not the case everywhere in the world today. In fact, even within the same society, plenty of people prefer a fuller figure. Thankfully, physical attractiveness can come in all shapes and sizes.

However, the media propagate an image of physical perfection that hugely influences how we judge our own physique. Never mind that more and more of the role models we see on screen and in magazines have been surgically "enhanced" and airbrushed to attain their look. We buy into these images and try to emulate them.

This often leads to feelings of frustration and inadequacy. These celebrities don't really look like that in the flesh in any case—certainly not first thing in the morning or last thing at night anyway! Second, we are all different and cannot be shoehorned into a one-size-fits-all ideal. The explosion of social media and filters that manipulate people's appearance is hugely detrimental to our self-esteem. It's as if the response to criticism of magazines for presenting these tampered-with images of supposed perfection has been to extend that ability to whole new generations—which now focus their attention on creating and disseminating faked photos of how they want to look rather than how they actually look. It's an ever-growing problem, especially for young girls. Indeed, the number of girls and women aged between 10 and 24 committing suicide in England and Wales has risen by 94 percent since 2012.

Dissatisfaction with appearance is a ticking time bomb for Generation Z (classed as those born between 1997 and 2012). It's not just phony photographic filters they're resorting to, but also cosmetic procedures such as lip fillers and full-blown cosmetic surgery even in their teens.

The desire to attain a beautiful body or shed a few pounds is one of the most common reasons for wanting to exercise. The principle is very simple: burn off more calories through exercise than you consume in food and drink, and you will lose weight, tone up, and look the way you want to look.

There are plenty of fitness regimes designed to help you do this. They seldom work for long because they never address the mental resistance to exercise, so the results are short-lived. The vast majority of people who go on an exercise regime to lose weight start to put it all back on again—and more—once they stop.

You cannot out-exercise a poor diet, or at least not forever. We all know people who were thin as a rake during their youth while consuming copious amounts of food, drink, desserts, cakes and pastries, but it all caught up with them later in life. The body can only take so much. It eventually gives up, leading to chronic weight gain.

EXERCISE FOR PERFORMANCE

Another reason for wanting to exercise is to be able to perform better. That can mean a whole range of things, from the person who just wants to feel more energetic or climb the stairs without getting out of breath to the athlete who wants to run faster, swim longer, compete better, etc.

As with exercising for appearance, there is a clear purpose, which can be tailored to achieve your goals. But again, it takes vast amounts of willpower to stick to your exercise regime, which makes the idea of not doing exercise seem precious—like a little treat. And as soon as you reach your goal, your motivation fades, the temptation to stop exercising takes over and you are back where you started.

Wouldn't it be great if we could all just maintain a comfortable fitness level without repeatedly putting ourselves through exercise plans? I have good news: you can. The key is do exercise as part of your routine without having to think about it, something that gives you pure enjoyment and fits into your lifestyle without being a big deal.

EXERCISE FOR CONSCIENCE

This brings me to the third big reason for wanting to exercise: the desire to feel good about yourself.

When you exercise, you always feel good about yourself afterwards. That is partly because you have achieved something that you wanted to do. It's also because the act of exercising releases hormones that make you feel happy. Remember the reward pathways in your brain? Exercise causes your body to release hormones that relieve pain, reduce stress, improve your wellbeing and happiness, and motivate you to do more exercise—a virtuous cycle.

Are you familiar with that feeling of relaxation, contentment and satisfaction that comes after exercise? It's a lovely sensation. Conversely, not exercising causes the opposite feeling. You are frustrated with yourself for ducking the challenge, you feel stuck in a rut, trudging through life, and you don't get the hormone boost, so your mood and self-esteem suffer.

WHY ANIMALS EXERCISE

Has it ever occurred to you that humans are the only creatures on earth that exercise for the reasons I have set out? When a dog is jumping up at the door because it's eager for its walk, is it really thinking, "Come on! I need my daily exercise, or I'll lose my figure!"? Wild dogs don't need to be taken for walks; they get exactly the right amount of exercise required for them to live healthily. It is only animals that rely on humans for their food or opportunities to exercise that don't automatically retain their natural health and vitality. Yet instinctively, they're still jumping at the door, looking forward to a good walk or run.

For dogs, as with all animals, exercise is instinctive. That includes humans. The problem is, it's an instinct we have lost touch with, as I will explain.

Wild animals get the exercise they need without having to plan it, promise themselves rewards or use self-discipline or willpower. For them, it is absolutely natural.

"Ah, yes," you might say, "but if wild animals didn't exercise, they would starve." True, they need to find their own food, whether they are a tiger or a dung beetle, and all that hunting and foraging keeps them as fit as they need to be.

Our ancestors had to hunt and forage too, and they were incredibly lithe and powerful—much stronger and fitter than we are today. They didn't go on diets or exercise regimes to reach the level of performance required to run down their prey. It was all part of a natural process.

Before you consign this book to the dustbin, I assure you I'm not suggesting you start foraging for your food! The point I'm making is that it's only modern humans, with our technological devices and automated lifestyles, who feel the need to force themselves through grueling exercise regimes.

For wild animals, there is a natural balance between sleep, movement, eating and the drive to forage. The exercise they take is a consequence of this balance. By following their instincts to eat and rest, other animals naturally get the exercise they need to stay in the shape they are designed to be. In fact, as mentioned already, it's only animals that have been domesticated by humans that suffer from a lack of exercise, overeating or both.

NATURE'S GUIDE

There is no need to live like prehistoric humans to appreciate how they naturally stayed fit as a result of their lifestyle. They instinctively knew that, in order to ward off hunger, they needed to go out to hunt or gather. As a result, they took regular exercise.

There must have been times when the effort was hard, but rather than thinking, "I need to keep running to beat my personal best," they must have thought, "I need to keep running or my family and I will not eat." Hunger was a powerful enough instinct to drive them through any pain barrier. It's the same for all animals because the need to eat is fundamental to survival.

Instincts are amazing. They're a survival guide, giving us all the signals we need to do the things we must in order to survive as a species. The same is true for all species. Every creature on earth follows this unwritten guidebook, which tells it when to move, rest, eat, run, hide, mate, etc.

I call this Nature's Guide. It works like a charm—when you let it. The problem for humans is that we have largely abandoned Nature's Guide. We go against our instincts. For example, we eat when we are not hungry; starve ourselves when we should eat; shun healthy foods in favor of junk that makes us overweight and lethargic; don't sleep when we are tired; and we consume addictive poisons like alcohol, nicotine and other drugs. All these abuses are threats to our existence and contrary to Nature's Guide. We would never do any of them if we simply followed our natural instincts.

BRAINWASHING

Why have we abandoned Nature's Guide when every other species in the world continues to follow it successfully? It's the same reason why human beings have become the dominant species on the planet: our intellect.

Intellect operates independently from instinct and is often in direct conflict with it. Our intellect has given us enormous advantages over the rest of the animal kingdom. It has enabled us to share information, such as where the saber-toothed tiger might be hiding or where the best berries can be found. It has given us the ability to gather and analyze information to predict dangers and outsmart our prey and predators.

All the modern conveniences I mentioned at the beginning of this chapter are the fruits of our intellect. It is an incredible gift, and we should be thankful for it. But it has also led us astray. Intellect is not just a positive force; it enables one human being to lie to another, to threaten and bully, to con and coerce. Everywhere you look, you can find examples of human intellect being used in negative ways.

Take billboards, for example. Advertising is the practice of persuading people that they need or want something they most likely don't actually need or want. It preys on aspirations and vulnerabilities, which are both facets of human intellect, and everybody is a target.

Our ability to communicate is an incredibly powerful tool, and like most tools, it can be used for good or bad. Our ability to miscommunicate is unfortunately equally powerful. The fact that millions of people willfully use it for that purpose every day shows just how complex the human psyche has become. Conscience plays a role in our behavior, and so does the ability to salve our conscience by kidding ourselves that our motivations are sound when they are anything but. These peculiarly human traits play a major role in the motivation to exercise and the tendency to avoid it.

Wild animals don't have these complications, so they follow Nature's Guide without question. Why do we kid ourselves? Because we have been bombarded with brainwashing from the day we were born. We have been fed a completely false impression of the world and the recipe for happiness – as false as the airbrushed images of those celebrity role models who inspired today's young generations to produce those fake, filter-enhanced selfies.

In the next chapter, we will examine how human intellect has left us trapped on the sofa.

Chapter 4

TRAPPED ON THE SOFA

It's been a long time since our ancestors had to hunt and gather food to survive. Our modern lifestyle is full of conveniences designed to save us from spending energy unnecessarily. However, this overlooks the fact that we are designed to spend energy, and if we don't, we become trapped in a miserable cycle of ill health and lethargy.

So far, I have given you two instructions: 1. Follow all the instructions. 2. Open your mind. You may already regard yourself as an open-minded person. The fact is, we all go through life with our minds largely made up by other people.

For example, when you see the sun rise in the morning, you understand that it appears to climb in the sky because the earth is turning. You don't see it as a fiery chariot being driven across the sky but as a ball of flaming gases burning millions of miles away. But how do you really know that is the case? Have you been to space and seen it for yourself? Or is it that you have been presented with very convincing arguments by people you regard as experts in that field, and their explanation tallies with what you see with your own eyes?

Don't worry, I'm not about to tell you that the earth is flat or the sun is a fiery chariot. The purpose of this book is to dispel myths. My point is that most of our knowledge is second-hand. Nevertheless, once we have been convinced, it takes a mental shift to make the human mind think differently. We tend to believe what we are told and once we do, it requires a change of perspective to believe something different.

So, why do we think of exercise as being hard? Sure, some exercise can be extremely grueling, but that sort of thing is usually reserved for athletes. It's actually easy for the average person to do regular, beneficial exercise that is not painful or hard at all.

Nor should it be. A dog doesn't run because it has to, it runs because it wants to. The same is true of young children. As soon as they are let out of class at break time, they rush around the playground, laughing and shrieking with joy. There is no pain involved. It's pure pleasure.

Give a bunch of kids a football or even a tennis ball, and they'll kick it around for hours. We were all like that once. And the fact that we're no longer like that has nothing to do with getting older, it has everything to do with us adopting unhealthy lifestyles as we age.

So why do we find it hard to exercise? Could it be because we have been brainwashed to believe that it is?

"No pain, no gain."

"Feel the burn."

These fitness mantras create the impression that unless you're pushing yourself through a pain barrier, then you might as well not bother. This is a hugely damaging message. It creates a negative attitude towards exercise that prevents many people from even attempting it, let alone sticking to it.

When children run around the playground, they are not thinking, "I've got to run for the next 10 minutes." They are running because instinct is driving them. When we are young, we enjoy a virtuous circle of motivation and exercise. We are motivated to play for pleasure, and exercise is a form of play. The exercise makes us feel good and we are galvanized to continue until we feel exhausted. The result is pure happiness. Watch children on the beach, by the pool or in the park. They love rushing around all day and have to be cajoled back home. As adults, we wonder where they get all that energy from.

At no time are they thinking about the exercise they are taking. They don't have to psych themselves up to run around the playground. It's the most natural thing in the world. Only when we stop and think about exercise do we start to think of it as a chore.

Professional football players are very fit. The average professional footballer runs more than six miles during a match, which lasts around 90 minutes. Much of that will be sprinting, and yet they barely notice the effort they are putting in. But tell them to go on a six-mile training run and prepare yourself for a chorus of grumbling.

So, what's the difference? When a footballer runs six miles during a game, their mind is occupied by the game itself. They have to think about their position, how they interact with their teammates, what the opposition is doing, where the ball is, what the manager is telling them, etc. The running they do occurs instinctively and automatically.

When a footballer runs six miles in pre-season training, they have none of those distractions to occupy their mind. The focus is all on the running. They start to notice the burning in their muscles, their breathing becomes heavy and fatigue sets in. The running ceases to be instinctive and becomes a conscious process.

When you exercise purely for the sake of what you want from exercise (better appearance, performance, etc.), your mind will focus on every ounce of effort much more than if you were doing something else at the same time. This is why gyms have TVs and loud music playing. It helps to take your mind somewhere else.

THE VOID

How and why do we lose that youthful enthusiasm that once sent us running around the school playground? Why do we come to regard running and other forms of exercise as a chore?

We talk about "the innocence of youth," and when you think about it, the way our mindset changes as we grow up seems to be largely about turning away from the things that are good for us and being drawn to things that we know are bad for us: alcohol, nicotine, cannabis and other drugs, gambling, late nights, etc.

"Wait a minute, that sounds like a recipe for a good night out!"

We joke about these things and like to think we can build them into our lives in moderation. But we also know they are damaging to our physical and mental health. Because we like a little excitement in our lives, we find the risk element of these things appealing. Not all the damaging behaviors we pick up later in life are exciting. We are also often drawn to working too hard and not making enough time for ourselves to relax and unwind.

So why do we abandon the healthy pursuits that we are drawn to instinctively and enjoy as children in favor of the unhealthy ones that control us and cause us problems as adults?

From the moment we are born, we seek security. It's like a void that we are constantly trying to fill. We instinctively reach for our parents for protection. This neediness continues through childhood when we are cocooned from the harsh realities of life in a world of make-believe. Sooner or later, though, we find out that Father Christmas and the Tooth Fairy don't exist, and the void returns.

At the same time, we are pushed from the safety of home into school, exposing us to new fears and insecurities. How good am I? How do I compare to my classmates? Who are my friends? What are the rules? What if I break them? All these uncertainties feed the void, and we seek reassurance to fill it.

As we enter adolescence, we start to look more critically at our parents and notice that they are not the unshakable pillars of strength that we had always assumed them to be. They have weaknesses, frailties and fears, just as we do.

This realization increases the void and as we become disillusioned and insecure. We unconsciously seek to fill the void with idols: pop stars, film stars, TV celebrities, sports players, etc. We create our own fantasies. We idolize mere mortals and try to absorb their reflected glory. Instead of becoming complete, strong, secure individuals in our own right, we become followers, impressionable fans, leaving ourselves wide open to suggestion.

Faced with all this confusion and insecurity, we look for a little boost now and then. Now, the brainwashing can really take hold. We are fooled into believing that alcohol and other drugs will generate the good times we need, that they will make us feel relaxed and happy, that they will give us status and help us to be accepted by our peers. So, we turn to alcohol or other drugs for relief from the void. Drugs such as cannabis and cocaine are more common than ever, and is it any wonder that young people get lured into trying them when so many TV series and movies feature them in a positive light? At our clinics, we address the damage done by these drugs and an important aspect of that damage is that they almost inevitably lead to a complete absence of exercise.

As we are drawn towards illusory props, we are pulled away from the beneficial pursuits of our childhood. We tire ourselves out with late nights and stress, eat junk food which saps our energy further, and end up trapped on the sofa.

These are all lifestyle choices we appear to make freely for ourselves, but they are based on misinformation. If we knew that alcohol would never actually make us genuinely happy, relaxed or confident, would we start drinking? If we knew that junk food doesn't actually taste good or give us any nutrition, would we start eating it? If we knew that spending hours on the sofa doesn't help us relax, but has the opposite effect, would we do it?

Please open your mind. Many of the lifestyle choices we appear to make as we grow up are based on brainwashing.

THE OBESITY MARKET

Choosing to eat junk food is an intellectual process, not an instinctive one. That means it's a decision you make based on acquired knowledge rather than instinct. Please don't assume that all "intellectual" decisions are clever. We've corrupted our taste buds so dramatically that we've forgotten how spectacular fresh fruit and vegetables taste. Even when we do eat them, we often smother them in sauces that eradicate their delicious natural flavors.

You may have been brainwashed into thinking that a Big Mac tastes better and is more satisfying rather than nutritious, delicious, natural food that keeps you healthy and in great shape.

If you were in touch with your natural tastes, you would find there is very little to excite the senses when it comes to junk food.

If we based our eating choices on our senses alone, we wouldn't touch it. So why do we consume it at all? Here are the arguments commonly put forward by the people who market junk food:

It's fast.
It's convenient.
It's cheap.
It tastes great.

These arguments are enough to convince us to eat junk food, even though it's no secret that it's not good for us. The lack of nutritional value doesn't bother us. Similarly, the known health risks of eating too much refined sugar, processed carbs and salt don't stop us. As long as we keep it in moderation, we assume we will be all right.

There's that word "moderation" again.

How many people succeed in keeping their consumption of junk food under control? The world is in the grip of an obesity epidemic, and it's only getting worse. According to the World Health Organization (WHO), worldwide obesity figures have almost trebled since 1975. Globally, two in every five adults aged 18 or over are overweight. More than one in eight are obese. And we are passing the problem on to our children in even greater numbers. That's quite aside from them becoming ever more sedentary and far removed from the kind of active childhoods we had prior to Gen Z.

Moderation has gone out the window for more than 2 billion people.

Another global health epidemic is type 2 diabetes, once known as "adult-onset diabetes" because, unlike type 1, it usually comes on later in life and is invariably caused by a poor diet and a lack of exercise. Today, type 2 diabetes is becoming increasingly prevalent among younger people. The total number of people with diabetes has quadrupled since 1980, and over 90 percent of cases are type 2. The WHO predicts that diabetes will be the seventh leading cause of all deaths worldwide by 2030.

Yet, all is not lost. It has been proven that simply by changing our diet, we can reverse not only pre-diabetes but also full-blown type 2 diabetes itself. Based on feedback from our "Good Sugar, Bad Sugar" program, in most cases, it takes less than a week or two. What's the secret? Remove junk food, refined sugar, processed carbs and replace them with real food. Imagine that… freedom from a lifetime of medication and risk of amputation, organ failure and blindness simply by ditching the junk!

JUNK FOOD IS LITERALLY KILLING US

It's also having a big impact on our attitude to exercise. Eating junk affects your willingness to exercise in two ways. First, it pricks your conscience and makes you want to exercise to make up for the junk you have eaten. Second, it makes you lethargic and less inclined to do the exercise you need.

This creates a conflict in your mind, a mental tug of war. It adds stress to the equation, which creates further conflict because stress also diminishes your willingness to exercise, while heightening your anxiety over not exercising.

We will examine this conflict in more detail later. For now, I want you to begin to see how lifestyle choices like the food you eat and the drugs you consume (including alcohol and nicotine) contribute to your aversion to exercise. You can reverse this situation by reversing your thinking about your lifestyle choices. You don't need to quit alcohol or nicotine to succeed. You do need to open your mind, question your beliefs and start seeing things in a different way.

ILLUSIONS

Brainwashing comes at us from many directions. Some of it comes from our parents and friends, some from our role models and a lot from advertising. Remember, the role of advertisers is to convince us that we want or need things that we neither want nor need. They do that by presenting products in a way that creates a subconscious connection between the product and the life we want to lead.

"Drink this and you'll have fun."

"Feed this to your kids and you'll get smiles all around."

"Wear this perfume and you'll be irresistible."

"Stick this in your mouth and inhale it, and you'll appear sexy."

It's laughable when you write it down in those terms, but advertisers do such a good job of dressing up their products that we become utterly convinced by these messages, often at a subliminal level. We unconsciously take their messages on board and don't stop to question them. Why would we? Everybody else seems convinced. When you do stop to question the brainwashing, you begin to see through the illusions. This is why opening your mind is so important. Without an open mind, you will continue to be fooled by the brainwashing.

Here is an illustration of the point. Take a look at the three different-sized people over the page.

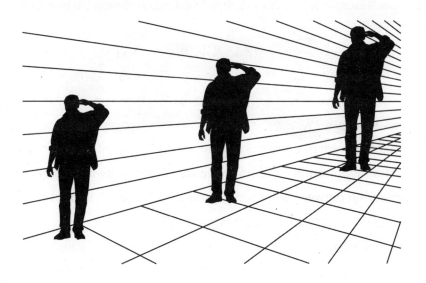

If I told you that the people in this drawing are exactly the same size, you would dispute that, wouldn't you? They all look different sizes, but that is because I told you they were different sizes and because of the way they have been presented. It's very easy to trick the human mind with imagery. Film directors do it all the time.

The fact is, these people are all identical. Take a ruler and measure them.

This illusion demonstrates how our minds can easily be tricked into accepting false "facts." As you continue through the book, remember this diagram and keep an open mind so that even if I tell you something that you find difficult to believe, you will at least accept the possibility that it might be true.

Let's look at another example. What do you think this says?

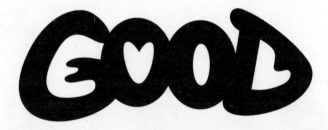

Now hold the book further away. Some people see the word "evil" to begin with but then see the word "good". Sometimes it's the other way around. Whichever way you see it first, once you're aware of both words, you can no longer convince yourself that there's only one. Can you see how easy it is to see the same thing in the opposite way when you're given a different perspective?

NEGATIVE ATTITUDES

A consequence of the brainwashing that we are subjected to throughout life is that not only do we fall for things that are bad for us, but we also develop negative attitudes towards things that are good for us.

These attitudes usually start during our teenage years and become ingrained in our twenties. Nutritious food, sleep, exercise, reading, quiet contemplation… as young adults, we tend to shun all these things as we embrace what we perceive to be the "good things in life." It's only later that we begin to understand how important these things are by which time we are so deeply conditioned against them that we find them hard to attain.

It's time to reverse that conditioning. This is an exciting moment in your life. The journey you are taking will be transformative. You are reading this book because you were unhappy about a particular aspect of your life: your struggle with exercise. It's time to banish the frustration and misery that comes with your inability to overcome your problem. You are holding the key to your freedom.

As you absorb this book, your mindset will determine how successfully you take in the information presented. An open mind is essential. A positive mindset is just as important.

THIRD INSTRUCTION: BEGIN WITH
A FEELING OF EXCITEMENT

You may feel trapped on the sofa, but that is about to change. You are going to rediscover the pleasure of exercise and the benefits will be life-changing.

Chapter 5

THE TRAP

I have compared your struggle with exercise to being in a trap. Let's take a close look at this trap and how it works. Once you can understand the nature of the trap you are in, escape becomes easy.

Traps work by luring their prey with bait and giving them the confidence to venture within beyond the point of no return. Think about a mousetrap or a lobster pot. Would the victim venture into the trap if they were aware of the danger?

Until the moment when the trap snaps shut, the victim is oblivious to this danger. But it has already been trapped and unless it somehow manages to escape, it will inevitably succumb.

The trap you're in works in the same way. Until you reach the point where you realize you are trapped, you remain oblivious to it. The purpose of this book is to enable you to understand the trap so that you can escape immediately. Don't worry if you fear you've left it too late. I have only good news for you. Your prognosis is wonderful, regardless of whatever shape you're in or your age.

THE PITCHER PLANT

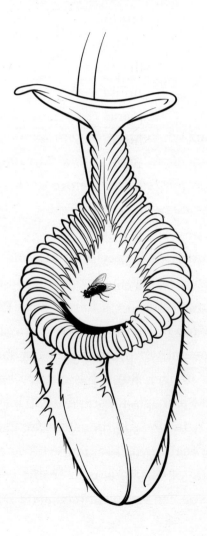

The pitcher plant offers a perfect illustration of falling for an illusory pleasure, with catastrophic results. This carnivorous plant, shaped like a tall, slender jug, catches flies with an ingenious and fatal confidence trick. The fly lands on the rim of the plant, attracted by the sweet smell of nectar. As it starts to feed, it doesn't realize that it is being lured further into the plant. The nectar tastes like the best thing in the world, but it is luring the fly to its doom.

The further down into the plant it slides, the steeper and more slippery the sides become until the fly can no longer hang on and falls into the belly of the plant, where a pool of digestive juices makes a meal of the poor thing.

In the last chapter, I explained why we are attracted to things that are bad for us. In trying to fill the void in our lives, we lap up the brainwashing and pin our faith in false pleasures like alcohol, nicotine, junk food, so-called recreational drugs and late nights. At this point in our lives, we are like the fly landing on the rim of the pitcher plant. We have a choice: we can fly away or continue to gorge ourselves on the nectar.

The brainwashing comes from people we trust, who themselves have been brainwashed by people they trust. It also comes from tricksters, whose job is to con us into making choices that contradict Nature's Guide. There is nothing natural about the position you find yourself in. Your aversion to exercise is not natural. We are designed to enjoy exercise, remember those children running around in the playground? It is a fabricated aversion created by brainwashing.

The brainwashing must be incredibly powerful because, as well as being attracted to these false pleasures, we also know very well that they present a variety of dangers. We know about the health risks associated with drugs and junk food. We know about the physical and mental torment of addiction. We know that the things we believe to be pleasures are also threats, but we trust our luck - "It won't happen to me."

Our confidence comes from seeing millions of other people who seem to be able to drink or smoke or eat what they want without apparently suffering any such problems. They are all in the same trap. Many of them sense that all is not well, but don't admit it, even to themselves. They want to believe that they are in control, so they try to bury any signs that that's not the case. They are in denial.

Be under no illusions, the world is full of people struggling like you, and for all of them, the struggle is caused by the same thing: brainwashing.

We try to con ourselves will be OK, that we will be one of the lucky ones. We disregard the harmful effects of our lifestyle choices, telling ourselves we are in control and can handle it.

In the early stages, everything seems to go OK. Nothing bad seems to be happening other than making yourself ill when you overdo it, which you just put down to inexperience. In fact, even if you repeatedly vomit in your early days of drinking, it just becomes par for the course. Your confidence is supreme, just like the fly on the rim of the pitcher plant, but without making a conscious decision, your consumption increases. You ignore warning signs, dismissing them as "normal."

YOU'RE ALREADY LOSING CONTROL.

As time passes, and the pleasure or comfort you seek to fill the void grows ever more elusive, you begin to sense that you are not in control. You are slipping further and further into a bottomless pit. It's an unhappy, insecure feeling that creates further anxiety and stress.

By now, you have conditioned yourself to seek relief from bad feelings like anxiety and stress by indulging in false pleasures like alcohol, other drugs or "comfort eating." You can see how this becomes a vicious circle of apparent need, fix, withdrawal, need… and as you're compelled to keep increasing the dose, the highs become more short-lived, the lows more intense. The net effect is an increasingly rapid descent, just like the fly sliding into the belly of the pitcher plant.

That is how the trap works. It's how any addiction works.

Let me reassure you again. I'm not saying you have to stop drinking, taking other drugs or go on a diet. I am saying that it will help you enormously to understand how these factors impact your desire and ability to exercise.

If you drink alcohol or smoke weed most days, think about whether you do so out of choice.

How did a glass of wine in the evening with dinner turn into a glass beforehand, another with dinner, and another after that? The same goes for weed. When did you decide that you'd take it every single day? Do you feel awkward or unsettled if, for any reason, you can't have that drink or joint in the evening? Perhaps you might run out, or someone wants you to pick them up in the car later in the evening. Or do you go out of your way to ensure that you never run out and avoid anything that might interfere with your evening tipple or toke?

Does your diet consist almost entirely of starchy and processed carbs (e.g. bread, pasta, pizza, pastries, etc), refined sugar (sweets, desserts, cookies, chocolate, ice cream, sugary drinks), and other processed foods (ready-meals, packet, tinned or bottled sauces)? Not one of the items above is natural food for human beings. And they are all nutritionally bankrupt. In fact, the only nutritional value lies in any vegetables, fruits, nuts or seeds that might be contained in them. That's why you can eat so much pizza or pasta. Your body is after the nutrition in the tomatoes and other vegetables that might be in the dish and continues to send you hunger signals until it has received enough of them. Hence the now well documented state of being "stuffed yet starved". Stuffed with junk but starved of the nutrients in natural foods.

Do you skip on sleep, sitting up late at night watching a screen? You need between seven and nine hours of sleep a night. Less can be highly detrimental to your energy levels and overall wellbeing.

Have a think about how many of the factors above in italics relate to your own life and consider their impact on your exercise problem.

ADDICTS SEEK COMFORT IN THE VERY THING THAT'S CAUSING THEM MISERY

You know that if you can just get into a routine of doing regular exercise, you will feel happy, healthy and good about yourself. Yet when you have the opportunity to exercise, too often you choose an alternative. For some reason, it seems more attractive at that moment, but afterwards it leaves you feeling unhappy, unhealthy and disappointed in yourself. Yet the same thing keeps happening over and over again. Why? Because you are in a trap.

A CONDITIONED RESPONSE

It's a clever con trick that fools intelligent, logical people into thinking that they get something positive from behavior that traps them in a vicious spiral of apparent need, followed by temporary relief, disappointment and emptiness, leading back to apparent need. I say "apparent need" rather than "need" because you never genuinely need these addictive drugs or behaviors, you are tricked into believing that you do.

With drug addiction, it's the chemical effect on the brain that causes this vicious spiral. When the drug is taken, you experience temporary relief from withdrawal from the previous fix, but the drug again leaves the body, causing a restless, niggling feeling, like an itch you can't scratch. When you decide to "let yourself off" exercising, you experience a similar momentary boost followed by a hollow, disappointed feeling. This feeling is partly mental disappointment at failing to live up to your own expectations and partly physical.

The momentary boost is caused by hormones being

released in the brain and forming a connection in your reward pathways. Remember, these pathways have an important role in encouraging us to do things that are good for us as a species. Exercise, sex and eating all cause these hormones to be released, and the feeling we experience incentivizes us to keep doing them. It's a simple and ingenious survival mechanism. Addictive foods, drugs and drinks interfere with this process. When the addictive substance is taken, the feeling of chemical withdrawal is momentarily relieved and you do feel better than a moment before, so the brain mistakes the substance for something that causes genuine, rather than phony, pleasure. Even that fake pleasure is fleeting, before the process of physical withdrawal begins again. It is in this way that addiction is like wearing tight shoes for the relief of taking them off.

When the boost is caused by deciding not to exercise—a decision you make because you believe you are choosing the more pleasurable option —it has a similar effect on the reward pathways as taking a drug. The boost is quickly replaced by a feeling similar to withdrawal, which creates an empty, restless feeling and sense of disappointment. How do you feel physically and mentally while gorging on pizza? How long after finishing it do you start to feel bloated, heavy, lethargic and guilty?

As more and more becomes known about the effects of the body's natural chemicals on the brain, the science confirms what we have been saying at Easyway for over 40 years. In 2019, Professor Robert West, one of the world's leading academics in the field of nicotine addiction, said this:

> "Nicotine causes dopamine release by nerve cells in the *nucleus accumbens*, a part of the brain involved in learning to do things. The dopamine release tells the brain to pay attention to the situation and what the smoker was just doing—and to do the same thing the next time they're in that situation. So, a link is forged between the impulse to smoke and situations in which smoking normally happens."

Professor West went on to add, "Crucially, the smoker doesn't have to feel any pleasure or enjoyment for this to work."

Now apply this to your decision not to exercise. You may not be conscious of any great boost each time you make that decision, but you have conditioned your brain to follow the same pattern when you think about exercising.

This conditioning dictates that when you consider doing exercise, an impulse *not* to exercise is simultaneously triggered. Without realizing it, you have become trapped in a vicious circle that controls you subconsciously. Every time you make the decision not to exercise, you reinforce the conditioning, making it more and more unlikely that you will make a different decision next time.

THE ILLUSION OF PLEASURE

All you are trying to achieve when you decide not to exercise is to regain the feeling of peace, calm and relaxation that you enjoyed before this vicious circle took control of you. But every time you make that decision, you guarantee that you will not feel peaceful, calm and relaxed; you will feel agitated and inadequate.

Avoiding exercise tends to be followed by feelings of guilt, shame, frustration and disappointment. The response is often to look for a pick-me-up. The temptation is to indulge in false pleasures that appear to give a temporary high, but these only compound your problem.

An alternative is to make a bigger effort next time, to try to assert greater control and force yourself to exercise. This struggle for control can be just as destructive. It requires tremendous willpower, which is not a recipe for enjoying regular exercise for the rest of your life. When your willpower runs out, the loss of control feels like a big blow, which adds to the negative emotions.

Easyway removes negative emotions from the equation. Exercise should be fun. The goal is to rediscover genuine pleasures that create lasting positive emotions. There are many wonderful, safe, healthy and non-addictive ways to stimulate the release of feel-good hormones for entirely positive effects. Many of them cost nothing: listening to music, dancing, cuddling, holding hands, laughing, carrying out a random act of kindness, making love… Fortunately, the list is endless.

These activities trigger a hormone release and leave you feeling genuinely happier in a way that lasts and is not quickly replaced by withdrawal symptoms. We allow genuine pleasures to be obscured by our pursuit of false pleasures. By now, you should know why: brainwashing.

Unraveling the brainwashing will help you reconnect with genuine pleasures, genuine sensations and genuine sources of contentment.

The "high" that we associate with nicotine, alcohol, and other addictive drugs is relief from the discomfort of withdrawal (the physical craving) coupled with relief from the mental feeling of deprivation caused by the illusion that the drug provides a genuine pleasure or comfort.

The same applies when you make the decision not to exercise. You are not choosing pleasure; you are choosing the illusion of pleasure.

Spending too much time at "Sofa Central" leaves you feeling lethargic, guilty and dissatisfied. It's like eating a box of chocolates. You might argue that it's possible to enjoy one or two chocolates, but you would never seriously suggest that scoffing down an entire box is enjoyable. How would that make you feel? Embarrassed, ashamed, awful, regretful, guilty and upset with yourself. And that's ignoring the physical effects! The same thing happens when you become a "Couch Slouch." Getting rest, relaxing and putting your feet up is fine—just not all the time.

Some people understand the point about fake pleasures but ask whether it really matters that the pleasure is fake. If it *feels* like pleasure, isn't that good enough?

It's a reasonable question. If we can be utterly taken in by the illusion of pleasure, does it matter that it's an illusion? You already know the answer to that. The perceived "pleasure" is fleeting and is quickly replaced by negative emotions. Indeed, when you make the decision not to exercise, you know deep down that it is not a choice that will leave you feeling good. What kind of pleasure leaves you feeling worse? Wouldn't it be better to replace it with genuine, lasting happiness?

CHANGING YOUR MINDSET

We've known for a long time that people can be brainwashed by bombarding them with propaganda. Tyrants have used this technique with devastating effect throughout history. It's only recently, however, that we have begun to understand why we are so susceptible to brainwashing.

Scientists have discovered that the brain is very plastic— meaning it can be molded and remolded by conditioning. Think of it as a network of electrical connections that fire off whenever you have a thought, process information, or pull something out of your memory. This network is continually changing shape to give more capacity where it is needed and less where it is not.

If you are given a large amount of information on one particular subject, the network will remold itself to accommodate this information. This happens when people become experts in specific fields. It's also how we become addicted.

The brain's plasticity determines not only knowledge but also attitude and mindset. The brainwashing we are bombarded with is designed to make us believe that there is pleasure in things that do us only harm. Our task is to help you change that mindset. In a sense, you are rewiring your brain.

It was understanding this aspect of addiction that enabled me to apply Easyway not only to smoking but also to alcoholism and other drug addictions, as well as addictions that don't involve taking a drug, such as gambling and overeating. I admit I knew nothing about the physical workings of the brain when I discovered the method—it just made perfect sense from my experience as a nicotine addict—and it has been very interesting to see science confirm all the basic ideas which underlie Easyway.

There are smokers who have quit but still crave cigarettes years later. You probably know at least one. The same applies to people who quit alcohol or other drugs. Some poor souls go on craving their little crutch for the rest of their lives. This is because they have quit through sheer willpower and have not changed their mindset, so they continue to believe that drinking, smoking or whatever other drug they took gave them pleasure or comfort and, therefore, they feel deprived without it. This is the interesting thing about addiction: the physical withdrawal from the drug isn't the problem—it's extremely mild—it's the belief that the addict is missing out on something pleasurable when they quit that causes all the angst and discomfort.

Addiction is a subtle combination of physical withdrawal (a very mild, slightly empty, insecure feeling) and brainwashing (the belief that we get tremendous pleasure or benefit from the drug and that we'll be miserable without it). Once you understand and accept that the pleasure or comfort is an illusion, solving your problem becomes not only easy but also enjoyable.

You may have no such addictions, but if you believe that avoiding exercise amounts to choosing pleasure, then you are in a vicious circle mindset that will keep you trapped until you find a way to reverse it. The good news is you have already found a way: this book.

THE DIFFERENCE BETWEEN YOU AND THE FLY

As you descend into the trap and begin to sense that you're not in control when it comes to exercise, you realize that the physical effects are starting to show. You might be putting on weight, your skin is losing its glow, and you're getting out of breath more quickly... These physical effects add to your negative emotions.

You get into the futile cycle of trying to muster the willpower to regain control, forcing yourself to exercise and then running out of steam and relieving the misery by giving up on exercise altogether. Like the fly in the pitcher plant, you only realize you're trapped when you're well and truly out of control. But there is one crucial difference between you and the fly:

YOU CAN ESCAPE ANY TIME YOU CHOOSE.

The trap you're in is not physical. Unlike the fly, you are not standing on a slippery slope. Your prison is entirely mental. It's ingenious because you're your own jailer and the more you struggle, the tighter the bonds become. Fortunately, that is also the trap's fatal weakness. Because you are the one keeping yourself trapped, you also have the power to set yourself free. All you have to do is follow the instructions in this book.

The wonderful thing is that when you escape, you will recover completely. Without the mental and physical lows induced by your struggle to exercise, you will be able to start enjoying genuine pleasures again to the full. I'm not suggesting that life will be a bed of roses. There will always be ups and downs. What I am saying is that the highs will be higher and the lows not as low.

You have the power to set yourself free. The fact that you have fallen into the trap has nothing to do with any flaw in your character or personality. Like millions of other people in the same situation, you have been brainwashed, until now.

DEBILITATING MYTHS

There are two major myths keeping you in the trap:

1. The myth that avoiding exercise gives you pleasure and/or comfort.

2. The myth that exercising involves hardship.

If you continue to believe these two myths, you will find it hard to change. No matter how desperately you *want* to, part of your brain will be telling you that you will be happier if you don't. We need to change your mindset. We need to unravel these myths.

We are conned into believing that avoiding exercise and chilling out instead gives us pleasure and comfort. Get it clearly into your mind, no genuine lasting pleasure or comfort can be gained from avoiding exercise. Quite the opposite.

Yet part of your brain will still be telling you that avoiding exercise is the easiest option, and you might be thinking, "Does it matter that it isn't true if it feels like it is?" There are two powerful arguments that should answer that question once and for all.

1. Avoiding exercise is a threat to your physical and mental health, and, if you go on burying your head in the sand, these grim realities will take their toll.

2. If you were happy about avoiding exercise, you would not be reading this book.

For the fly in the pitcher plant, there is a point at which it senses it's trapped and tries to escape. It is always too late. The fly struggles a bit, loses its footing and falls into the digestive juices.

For you, though, it is different. The trap you are in is entirely mental. So, when you sense that you are being consumed by your struggle with exercise and want to become free, there is no physical barrier to stop you. You know there is no genuine pleasure, no comfort, no reason at all to avoid exercise. From this strong foundation, it is a short step to establishing the mindset you need to walk free.

The illusion of pleasure makes it hard for people to change their mindset. Once the illusion of pleasure is gone, there is only one thing holding you back:

FEAR

It's an odd kind of fear—the fear that escaping from a miserable situation will leave you feeling even more miserable—but it's genuine , and we will tackle it very soon. First, though, we need to look more closely at the illusion of pleasure and the myths that keep controlling your mind.

Chapter 6

FIRST STEPS TO FREEDOM

The mindset that keeps you in the trap is built on the illusions of false pleasures. Now that you are aware of the trap, you can start to see through these illusions and change your mindset.

If you have been trying for years to overcome your struggle with exercise—as millions of people do—you might just be hoping to miraculously wake up transformed into a "sporty person" who exercises on a regular basis and enjoys every minute of it.

You may be reading this book because you heard that Easyway works like magic and want to know the secret. You might even feel frustrated that I haven't just told you the magic formula and sent you away to get on with it.

Before we go any further, it's important that you understand two things:

1. There is no secret.

2. There is no magic.

Many people who have escaped their addictions with the help of Easyway have spoken about its effectiveness as if it were a miracle cure because it makes the process of becoming free so easy and enjoyable and the benefits are so wonderful. Easyway itself however, is based on strict logic and reason and that is why it is so effective—because it makes complete sense. There is no leap of faith, no complex science, no demands on your concentration or willpower. As you take on board the reasoning, you will form a clearer and clearer understanding of the trap you are in and the way to escape from it, just as a distant object comes into focus as you walk towards it.

By using logic, Easyway strips away the illusions put into your mind by brainwashing and replaces them with clear, rational thought, which removes your desire for false pleasures. The key is the set of instructions you receive throughout the book, and it must be used like the combination lock of a safe. Each step must be understood and applied in the correct order for the combination to work.

You have already been given the first three instructions, and your escape plan is well under way, so please be patient. The key to your escape does not lie in the final chapter, the first chapter, or any single chapter alone. The whole book is the key.

THE ILLUSION OF CHOICE

Who forces you to choose not to exercise? Does anyone hold a gun to your head and order you to spend the evening on the sofa instead?

Perhaps you're not a "Couch Slouch" at all, in which case I apologize. Maybe you're always snowed under by work, don't get home until late, and barely have time to grab a bite to eat, let alone slob out in front of the TV. Or perhaps you're a single parent, spinning plates all day? Perhaps by the time you've got the kids to bed, done the household chores and all the other countless things you need to do, you deserve to put your feet up.

Whichever group you fall into, and although it might now seem impossible to think of a way to lighten your load enough to free up time to exercise, by the end of this book, you will be straining at the leash to get your body moving again and nothing will prevent you from doing so. In any case, something has to change or your body will give up. And you're no good to your business or your kids if that happens.

Whatever your circumstances, you end up not exercising. But is it really a choice? If it were, why would you keep making a choice that leaves you frustrated and miserable? Given the choice, wouldn't you rather exercise? Isn't that why you're reading this book?

The "choice" to avoid exercise is driven by the myths mentioned in the last chapter: that exercising is hard and that avoiding exercise gives you some sort of pleasure or comfort. The pleasure or comfort that you imagine you are choosing is an illusion.

In the last chapter, I explained how the mind becomes conditioned to avoid exercise by repeatedly making that choice. If you repeatedly choose not to exercise, your brain learns to see that choice as pleasure. This is because making that choice causes a momentary boost, which the brain remembers. So, when we talk about "choosing" not to exercise, you're not really making a choice at all; you're following a subconscious impulse that has become established over time.

This is a key point. The frustration you feel at not being able to "discipline" yourself enough to stick to a regular exercise regime is founded on the belief that you keep making "the wrong choice." So, you become annoyed with yourself, you decide to get tough with yourself and you dig into your reserves of willpower to force yourself to make the right choice.

But this punishing approach only lasts so long. It's not a formula for happily maintaining regular exercise for life. If anything, it is likely to put you off exercise forever.

When you recognize that it's not you making "the wrong choice" but the result of brainwashing that has conditioned you to behave the same way repeatedly, you can stop being so hard on yourself. Instead of punishing yourself by forcing yourself to exercise, you can address the situation with a clearer mind and approach it from a different angle.

FITS AND STARTS

The struggle with exercise is often characterized by binges and droughts. You go through cycles of throwing yourself into an exercise regime and then getting tired of it and not exercising at all. One state leads to the other.

When you're not exercising, you start to feel guilty and self-conscious. You notice that you're putting on weight and climbing the stairs isn't as easy as it was. When you begin exercising, those feelings of guilt and self-consciousness fade and your motivation to exercise fades with them. Without that motivation, you ask yourself whether you really need to keep going.

Drug addicts are the same. Smokers and drinkers are notorious for stopping and starting. They make a huge effort to stop but when they feel they have regained some degree of control, they reward themselves with a smoke or a drink. "Just the one; what's the harm?" The harm is that "just the one" is all it takes to re-trigger the addictive spiral they were so desperate to escape in the first place.

The trap works in the same way for everyone. It is characterized by a pattern of highs and lows, peaks and troughs. There are periods of "control," during which you might feel like you are being tough on yourself, interrupted by spells of "loss of control," where you think you are being easy on yourself, but which leave you feeling worse.

I put "control" in inverted commas because I'm not talking about genuine control. Genuine control is an easy, relaxed condition in which logic and truth lead to sound decisions being made without any great effort. The cycles of "control" and "loss of control" that happen in the trap are caused by the illusions that underpin it. They take you from one extreme to another. That is not control. That is confusion and chaos.

When you feel "the loss of control," it drags you down both physically and mentally. You don't get the exercise you need for your health, nor do you get the satisfaction from doing what you really want to do. When you re-establish "control," the guilt and disappointment go but are replaced by a feeling of deprivation and sacrifice. It's not a comfortable, natural state because you have to apply enormous willpower. At no point in this cycle are you truly happy.

So, how can you break free from it? First, you have to change the way you look at the problem. Instead of trying to control your impulse to avoid exercise and forcing yourself to do it, we need to remove that impulse altogether so that you can enjoy exercise and even look forward to it as the genuine source of pleasure that it really is.

This simple shift in attitude removes your mental conflict so that all your will is directed towards exercising, removing the need for willpower.

STAYING FREE

Imagine the trap like a hole in the ground into which you have fallen. Between us, we have the two essentials that will set you free: you have a strong desire to get out and I have the information that will enable you to do so. All you have to do is follow my instructions.

However, once you have escaped, there is a further danger: the trap still exists. We have to ensure that you do not fall back into it again.

We can do this by ensuring you understand the nature of the trap. Unlike a hole in the ground, the trap is not physical but psychological. It exists entirely in your mind. It is an illusion conjured up by brainwashing.

The trap is easy to fall into. Fortunately, it is just as easy to escape, provided you understand it. Look again at the illusion of the three figures on page 55. You were convinced that they were different sizes because of the way they were presented. It took the strict rationality of measuring them to dispel the illusion and understand that what you are seeing is not actually what is there. The visual trick is so effective here that even when we know that the figures are the same, they still look different. Now look again at the good / evil graphic in the same chapter. Once you have seen the word "evil", you will not be able to unsee it. This is how Easyway works. Once you have seen the truths behind the illusions you will not be fooled again.

The brainwashing we are all subjected to from birth has given us false impressions. These false impressions, coupled with the chemical effect in the brain that occurs when we pursue false pleasures, create the illusion of pleasure. When we believe in the illusion, it follows that we feel deprived and miserable if we deny ourselves that "pleasure."

So, what gain or payoff do you get when you "make the choice" not to exercise?

CHOOSING A MYTH

When you choose to "let yourself off" exercise, what do you do instead? Put your feet up? Curl up on the sofa? Watch TV? Read a book? Have a snack? A drink? These activities may be pleasures, but they take on a false quality as an alternative to exercise. At the back of your mind, you know that this isn't what you should be doing—a guilty pleasure. But it's not a genuine pleasure if there is an uncomfortable, conflicting thought eating away at you like a worm.

When you finish this book and conquer your acquired aversion to exercise, you will find that many "guilty pleasures" become genuine pleasures again which you are free to enjoy to the full without doubts or complications. You will find that your life regains the vitality and *joie de vivre* of those young children we see rushing around the park for the sheer joy of it!

Why would you choose any alternative to exercise when it leaves you feeling restless and dissatisfied? The answer is simple: you don't. You don't make this choice; you are conditioned to avoid exercise because of the way your mind has been affected by the brainwashing.

When you "choose" not to exercise, you believe that you are choosing pleasure over pain. You believe you are letting yourself off a hardship and choosing a more relaxing option. You are falling for the myths that exercise is hard and that the alternative will be pleasurable. It's time to dispel these myths once and for all.

If you believe in mantras like "No pain, no gain" or "feel the burn," you will naturally think exercise is difficult. Some so-called experts will tell you that it's not doing you any good unless it hurts. This is nonsense, and it's essential to understand how ridiculous this assertion is.

Going for a brisk walk is wonderful exercise. It works the heart, lungs and legs. It allows your mind to wander and unwind and gives you access to fresh air and sunlight. Is walking a grueling form of exercise? Of course not. It's gentle, relaxing and enriching.

Walking is just one example of the many ways you can give your body the exercise it needs without any hardship, mental struggle or financial cost. Many people get similar pleasure and benefits from cycling and swimming without ever having to push their limits. It is pure, easy enjoyment.

Anything that involves movement is good exercise. The belief that you have to push yourself through pain is a major obstacle to establishing a regular, healthy exercise pattern. At the same time, the belief that the alternatives are a greater source of pleasure is equally damaging. There is nothing wrong with spending an evening on the sofa, but it doesn't leave you with the sense of joy and satisfaction that comes from exercise, and if you're spending EVERY night on the sofa, it ceases to be enjoyable at all. Spending all of your spare time lounging around is like scoffing an entire box of chocolates—you're left feeling guilty, ashamed, out of shape and depressed.

We are designed to enjoy exercise because it is beneficial for our survival. The body releases hormones that make us feel genuinely good and genuinely better when we exercise. This doesn't happen when we are inactive. It doesn't happen when we eat junk food, take drugs, or drink alcohol. Remember, any gain in feel-good hormones in those circumstances is triggered by the temporary ending of the discomfort addiction causes. It's like taking two steps backwards and then one step forward. The hormones released by a genuine pleasure such as exercise, give you a giant leap forward. The choice to do nothing rather than exercise is not a choice for pleasure, it's not even a choice for the avoidance of pain; it is simply the choice to do nothing. Doing nothing is OK. In fact, it's good to do nothing from time to time, but it's not a long-term, full-time strategy for happiness.

You believe that you are choosing pleasure over pain when you choose to avoid exercise because you have been brainwashed. Remember I told you to keep an open mind and question everything? Well, now it's time to question everything you think you know about the choices you make as an alternative to exercise.

Ask yourself, "How good does this feel?" "Am I truly relaxed and happy?" "Is my mind at ease?" "Is this the way I want to spend the rest of my life?"

All your life, you have been fed misinformation about the things that give you pleasure. Now, you need to question that misinformation. "Is this really true, or have I been taken in by an illusion?" "Are those figures in the illustration really different sizes or are they the same size?"

By questioning your current beliefs, the truth will become clear. We are not often encouraged to question our preconceptions. We tend just to follow the flock. It's essential that you start thinking for yourself and questioning what you have, until now, passively accepted as true simply because society has brainwashed you.

In the next two chapters, we will look more closely at the flaw that connects all humans and how this can cause us to make bad choices. You will also learn how easy it is to overcome this flaw.

Chapter 7

THE INCREDIBLE MACHINE

*To get to the root of your aversion to exercise, we need to take
a moment to talk about Nature and our relationship with food.
If you're wondering what this has to do with exercise, please
remember the second instruction and keep an open mind.*

THE SQUIRREL

It's funny how the most everyday occurrences can trigger the most
important discoveries in our minds. Archimedes was stepping
into the bath when he had his "Eureka!" moment; Sir Isaac
Newton was inspired by an apple falling from a tree; for me, it
was a squirrel that drew my attention to Nature's Guide.

I always enjoyed watching the squirrels in my garden; their
agility was a constant source of wonder. My cat enjoyed watching
them too, albeit for different reasons. I marveled at how the

squirrels always seemed to know the cat was watching and were always too nimble to be caught.

On one occasion, I was watching a squirrel sitting on my patio, happily eating nuts. I thought to myself, "Eat too many of those and you won't be able to escape the cat!" As if it had read my mind, the squirrel immediately stopped eating the nuts and started burying them.

I couldn't stop wondering why the squirrel had chosen to stop eating when nuts were aplenty. If someone put a bowl of nuts in front of me, I would have scoffed them all. If I was foolish enough to eat until the food ran out, why wasn't the squirrel? Here was I, a member of the most intelligent species on the planet, being outsmarted by a mere rodent. It had to be about something other than intelligence.

Anyone can see the sense in saving some food for later, especially when you are a creature that can never be sure where your next meal is coming from. But how could the squirrel know that? How could an animal with a brain not much bigger than the nut it was eating have the foresight to stop eating when food was abundant and store some away for later?

More to the point, why didn't the squirrel have a weight problem? Did it know that if it overate, it wouldn't be able to escape the cat? This goes back to the point I made in Chapter 3 about animals being more or less uniform in size and weight. I realized that I had never seen a squirrel with a weight problem. In fact, I had never seen a wild animal of any species that was overweight.

Sure, there are animals like walruses and hippos that seem fat, but that's the shape that Nature intended. I have never seen a walrus or hippo that is distinctly overweight compared to the rest of the herd.

Think of the amazing images we see of animals in large groups. It could be a school of fish, a herd of water buffalo, a flock of geese. Their individual sizes may differ, but they're all the same shape and proportion. There are none that lag behind the others, weighed down by an oversized belly caused by overeating.

It dawned on me that human intelligence isn't the only thing that sets us apart from the animal kingdom. We are also the only species on the planet that has weight problems—we and the domesticated animals whose eating habits we control or animals like pigeons and vermin that scavenge on the junk food that humans cast aside as waste.

This was my "Eureka!" moment. It was an overwhelming piece of evidence: 99.99 percent of all the creatures on Earth eat as much of their favorite foods as they want, as often as they want, without being overweight. Obviously, there must be a simple secret, so simple that a squirrel could comprehend it. That secret is Nature's Guide—the instincts that help us survive.

NATURE'S WARNING SIGNS

The reason why the squirrel stopped eating the nuts was because it was no longer hungry. It sounds so incredibly simple, yet the most intelligent species on the planet can't seem to work it out.

Hunger is one of the many warning signs that Nature's Guide uses to keep us healthy and safe.

Sight, smell, hearing, touch, and taste all play a vital role in keeping us alive. Watch a wild animal when it approaches unfamiliar food. It won't dive in and start feeding immediately. First, it will scrutinize the food, perhaps circling it once or twice. Then, it will sniff it. If the food passes these tests, the animal will touch it suspiciously, always ready to walk away. Finally, it will taste it, testing a small morsel before tucking into the rest.

This is how Nature's Guide enables all animals to detect the best food for them. These senses are all any animal needs. It's an ingenious system and it works like a dream. Your senses do the same for you. You can tell when an apple is rotten just by looking at it. It might look edible if it's on the turn, but it will smell off and be soft to the touch. If you took a bite, the taste would be repugnant and you would spit it out. An experience like that might put you off apples for a while.

If you were to eat and drink the correct foods and liquids according to whether you feel hungry, you would be your ideal weight. Hunger is a direct signal that your body is low on nutrients, which in turn is directly related to the amount of energy you burn off (exercise). It can even create a desire for the specific foods you need for the nutrients you lack. There is no better indicator of the fuel your body needs.

We tend not to have a problem responding to hunger. The first pangs are enough to send us to the cookie jar. Where we do have a problem is responding to the absence of hunger—because when you no longer feel hungry, your body sends a signal, as with the squirrel, that you no longer need to eat.

But we don't stop eating when we are no longer hungry. We are conditioned to eat and drink at set times of the day and in set quantities, regardless of how much exercise we have had or our hunger gauge. Our intellect has designed a system that disregards our instincts—and look where it has got us!

The flaw in the incredible machine is that we put our faith in our intellect over our instincts. Because we don't understand our instincts, we regard them as hit or miss—nothing more than guesswork. But instinct is not hit or miss; it is the result of millions of years of trial and error. It is what enables wild animals to avoid eating anything harmful to them.

Humans, meanwhile, are brainwashed into consuming all manner of poisons: refined sugar, caffeine, alcohol, nicotine, etc. Perhaps the most obvious example of this brainwashing at play is during a child's birthday party. These events are always emotionally charged and usually, at least one child ends up sick. All that cake, mountains of cookies, candy, and chips, all those sugary drinks—children overdo it in their excitement, and they just can't keep it down. But have you ever stopped to wonder exactly why they are sick?

There are two important observations here:

1. Children do not naturally self-regulate when faced with an abundance of sugary food.

2. They don't just feel ill after eating it; they bring the food back up.

The first point is evidence that junk food, such as refined sugar, has very little nutritional value. This is well-known and generally accepted. The problem with food of very little nutritional value is that it hardly registers on the hunger gauge, so you continue to feel hungry even when your stomach is full. This is why, after eating an enormous pizza, you can still feel hungry for dessert. Junk has some of the characteristics of food, but it lacks the vital ingredients that the body needs, so it doesn't satisfy hunger, and children will keep eating it until they physically can't take any more.

The second point is evidence of another ingenious function of our bodies. We are built with a natural stomach pump for occasions when we poison ourselves. When your body detects poison, it does everything it can to expel it from your system. If you have ever experienced vomiting to the point where you feel there is nothing left to come up, you will know just how effective your body can be in clearing out poison. It's painful and unpleasant, but it's a lifesaver.

You might be questioning the suggestion that refined sugar is a poison. After all, we are not sick when we eat it in smaller amounts. The truth is that refined sugar gives you virtually no nutritional benefit whatsoever, and if you eat enough of it, it will always make you feel ill. But then, why are children drawn to refined sugar if it is so unhealthy? As a species, we are predisposed to like sweet foods because it allows us to detect the best sources of glucose in nature, i.e. fruits, which also happen to be full of nutrients, vitamins, and fiber. However, the food industry uses refined sugar to replicate the sweetness of fruit, and children are unable to tell the difference. Nor are adults.

The human body is not only fine-tuned to perform at its best when given the right fuel but is also incredibly resilient when given the wrong fuel. Compare it to a car. If you put diesel in a gasoline-powered engine, you will be lucky if it ever works again. At the very least, you will have an expensive repair on your hands. But when you eat the wrong foods, your body does its best to absorb the impact, even to the extent of developing a tolerance to the poison.

This is one of the amazing attributes of the human body, but it should not be taken for granted. Your body's capacity to roll with the punches is not infinite, and while there may be no physical signs of damage on the outside for a while, the damage on the inside can be severe. The body's resilience and brainwashing from the food industry have led us to believe we can get away with eating just about anything. But the statistics on obesity, diabetes, heart disease, and other ailments prove the opposite is true. It's time to recognize how incredible your body is and start treating it as the most precious thing in your life. Because that is exactly what it is… yet we barely give its care a second thought.

Now, what exactly do I mean when I talk about the "wrong food" or "junk?" Which are the "right foods" and how do we know? The answer is simple: the right foods are those that Nature's Guide tells us to eat.

YOUR FAVORITE FOOD

We have a very good understanding of the nutrients our bodies need to function. We know we must keep hydrated and consume a balanced diet that gives us vitamins, minerals, fiber, protein, carbohydrates, etc. Our ancestors didn't have this knowledge, so how did they stay fit and healthy? You guessed it—Nature's Guide. Why do you think certain foods taste better than others? Why is a glass of cool, clear water the best thing to quench your thirst on a hot summer's day? In fact, why do we have a sense of taste at all? Because Nature gave us all a tool to help us identify the right foods: taste.

THE FOODS THAT TASTE BEST ARE ALSO THE BEST FOR US

At this point, your jaw may have hit the floor. The foods that taste best also happen to be best for us. Really? Doesn't that go against what I've just been saying about sugary foods? Please keep an open mind—this is how you see through the damaging illusion that sugary foods taste best.

When you think of your favorite foods, you might well imagine a bar of chocolate or a piece of cake. Just like the children at the birthday party, we are brought up to regard these foods as treats and are brainwashed into thinking sugary "treats" are our favorite food and this is the food that tastes best. And then we are told not to eat too much of this type of food because it's not good for us. How confusing! We are conditioned to associate tasting good with being bad for us.

In other words, sugary junk food is given the mystique of forbidden fruit. So it's no surprise we yearn for it as children and indulge ourselves with it as soon as we are old enough to buy our own.

But have you ever actually paid attention to the taste in your mouth when you eat these foods? Or the way you feel afterward? Observe those children at the party table. Do they eat slowly? Do they savor each mouthful? No, they chow it down before they have properly chewed it. Next time you eat cake or a chocolate bar, pay attention to the taste, the smell, and the feeling in your mouth. You will realize that it is nothing special and may even find it revolting. Then, monitor how you feel afterward. You will notice a restlessness and a sense of agitation. That is the effect of refined sugar on your body and mind.

Now compare that to eating a crisp apple or a juicy piece of mango or any other delicious fruit for that matter… the aroma, the texture, the flavor, the after-feel. Humans love the taste of fruit. If you want proof, look at the food and drink at a children's party. It will mostly, if not entirely, be fruit flavored. Fruit is humans' favorite food, and it also happens to be the most nutritious food in our diet.

FREE YOURSELF FROM THE BRAINWASHING

Our relationship with food lies at the heart of our detachment from Nature's Guide. You can see the tragic results of this everywhere: weight issues, health issues, anxiety, and depression. You might think that if the brainwashing has been going on for so long, it will take a mighty effort to change. And if we have become so detached from our senses and instincts, how will we ever be able to reconnect? The good news is that your body has an incredible power to adapt.

DON'T BE A SLAVE TO YOUR CURRENT TASTES

Take tea or coffee, for example. Many people start out drinking tea or coffee with sugar and fear that if they were to cut it out, it would taste awful. However, after just a week or less of re-adjustment to having no sugar, if you were to give that person a cup of tea or coffee with sugar, they would react as if you'd given them poison. You could say they've un-acquired the taste for sugar in coffee or tea, or they've acquired the taste for coffee or tea without sugar. The point is their taste has changed completely and very quickly.

Eating nutritious food will significantly help to overcome your aversion to exercise. It will give you energy, reduce your susceptibility to lethargy, and reduce the amount of exercise you need to stay fit.

FOURTH INSTRUCTION: FOLLOW NATURE'S GUIDE AND FREE YOURSELF FROM SLAVERY TO YOUR PRESENT TASTES AND EATING HABITS.

Remember, keeping an open mind means questioning both sides of the argument. Until you complete this book and are convinced that everything I've told you is true, I want you to accept the possibility that it *could* be true—but I don't want you to accept it blindly. Question both sides of the argument. That is the way to arrive at the truth.

Chapter 8

HOW FIT DO YOU WANT TO BE?

The fact that you feel guilty when you don't exercise suggests that you regard exercise as something you <u>should</u> do rather than something you <u>want</u> to do. So, how much exercise do you think you should be doing?

According to the medical community, the recommended amount of exercise for anyone between 19 and 64 is 150 minutes of moderate exercise, or 75 minutes of vigorous exercise, per week. In addition, doctors advise you to do muscle-strengthening exercises at least twice a week.

Moderate exercise is any activity that raises your heart rate and makes you warm up, such as a brisk walk or a bike ride. Vigorous exercise is any activity that makes you breathe hard and fast, like running, cycling uphill, or playing sports such as football or tennis.

Doesn't that strike you as odd? Surely a 19-year-old and a 64-year-old need different amounts of exercise? And what about other variables like height, sex, or diet?

This recommendation aims to reduce the risk of heart disease and strokes. So, is that why you exercise? In Chapter 3, we looked at the three main reasons why people want to exercise:

1. To look the way they want to look.
2. To perform better.
3. To feel good about themselves.

Part of feeling good about yourself is knowing that you are doing something to protect your long-term health. Animals don't think "I must get on that treadmill or I'll increase my risk of getting heart disease," yet they remain the size and shape they need to be and have the energy they need to perform. Whether they feel good about themselves is hard to tell. What we do believe is that wild animals don't suffer from the mental anguish that humans do, such as self-loathing or suicidal thoughts. These are very human conditions—an unfortunate by-product of our intellect.

For other animals, exercise is not a conscious choice, it's automatic—a natural part of their everyday life. They don't question whether they are getting the hormone release they need; it just happens naturally. Imagine if you could make exercise a natural part of your life in the same way.

The good news is that you can. First, you must understand the relationship between exercise, consumption, and how you look and feel. For most humans, that relationship has been turned inside-out. Dissatisfaction with the way you look and feel creates a desire for types of food and drink that leave you looking and feeling worse (i.e. junk), so you force yourself to exercise to remedy the situation.

No wonder you have an aversion to exercise. Any remedy that requires such willpower is hardly a pleasure. As soon as your willpower gives out, the exercising stops. Then you are back to square one, feeling more miserable than before because another attempt to get on top of your health and fitness has failed.

So, let's examine this relationship and see how you can fix it for good.

TARGET WEIGHT

It's natural to care about your appearance. We all want to look in the mirror and be happy with what we see. But it can become obsessive, and one of the biggest obsessions associated with looking the way we want is weight.

If you are slimming down, it's natural to expect your weight to fall. If you are bulking up, you'll expect to see your weight rise. The problem arises when you set yourself a target weight. You may have looked at websites that claim to be able to tell you your ideal weight. Type in your height and gender and a weight or weight range pops up. If you have used one of these sites to find your target weight, please forget it.

Weight charts provide a marvelous excuse for anyone struggling to lose weight. They are made out to be scientific, but in reality, they are nothing of the sort. It is ridiculous to suggest that there is a simple equation that can be applied to everyone.

In our sugar-addiction and weight-loss seminars, asking the group to picture Usain Bolt is always interesting. What do you think Usain Bolt weighed when he was winning all those gold medals? The estimates we get vary by as much as 44 lbs (20 kgs)!

I never actually knew Usain Bolt's weight, and I doubt whether he knew it either. It was glaringly obvious that he was in superb physical condition and at the exact weight he wanted. If you were in a similar physical condition, would you care how much you weighed? Of course not.

The fact that estimates vary by 40-plus pounds emphasizes how unhelpful it is to set yourself a target weight. It shows that we actually have no idea about the correlation between what the scales tell us and what we see in the mirror.

Look at your friends. Do you need a set of scales to know which are overweight? Of course not. If you think you are overweight, did you come to that conclusion by looking at the scale? Or was it the sight of your reflection in the mirror, the fact that you felt short of energy, and that the slightest exertion left you out of breath?

Your scale will not tell you when you are the weight you want to be—your eyes and your lungs will. Your ideal weight is not some figure spewed out by a computer algorithm; it is the weight you are when you look at yourself in a full-length mirror and are happy with what you see. It is the weight you are when you wake up every morning bursting with energy. It has nothing to do with mathematics or guesswork.

The claim that exercise is essential to weight loss is another con. What happens when you exercise? You burn off more fuel, which increases your metabolism. But exercise also makes you hungrier, so you increase your intake.

RUNNING MAN

I knew a man in his 40s who decided to run the London Marathon. He was overweight and thought the exercise would help him shed some pounds and give him a sense of achievement. When he began training a year before the run, he weighed 240 lbs.

He was a disciplined man. Every day for 12 months, he put in the work and got up at 6 am to run for an hour before work. When the London Marathon finally came around, he completed the course in just over four hours.

Thrilled with his achievement, he rushed home and went straight to the bathroom to weigh himself. He had to laugh. The scale read the exact same weight as a year ago, before all the training and the marathon.

This didn't depress him as much as you might think because he already knew in his heart that he had not lost weight. He could feel it. For every ounce he had burned off jogging, he had eaten and drunk more to satisfy his increased hunger.

FUELING UP AND BURNING OFF

There is one simple reason why we put on or lose weight. You may ask yourself the question out of exasperation, but regardless of all the complicated advice surrounding diets, exercise, and willpower, the answer is very straightforward. A body will gain weight if you add more to it than you take away. This is the balance between intake and disposal that wild animals manage to maintain without even thinking about it.

Let's go back to the comparison between the human body (the incredible machine) and the car. Imagine if you decided for some reason that your car weighed too much. Would you take it out for a drive just to burn off some fuel? I'm sure you agree that would be crazy. But it is precisely what we do to our bodies when we use exercise regimes to lose weight.

If you regard exercise as something you need to do to lose weight, you are missing the fact that you must be over-fueling to put on weight in the first place. Over-fueling has become an epidemic among humans because of the type of fuel we consume.

Think about how you fuel your car. Do you follow the same routine as you do with eating and put in the same amount at the same time every day? What if you don't use the car for a week? Will you still go and put your usual amount in the tank? We all know what would happen if you did. There would be gas spilling out all over the driveway. This is exactly how we tend to fuel up our bodies: the same quantities at the same times every day, regardless of the hunger gauge. The junk sloshes into our midriff, buttocks, waist, chest, arms, legs, neck, and face and sits there in unsightly bulges.

We don't treat our cars this way because we are in no doubt that the manufacturer intended us to put fuel in the car for no other reason than to make it run—and we trust the fuel gauge. We understand the logic because the car was designed by humans and humans are the leading experts on how it works.

When it comes to the incredible machine, we lose sight of this simple logic because we have been brainwashed to fuel up according to a set routine rather than rely on Nature's Guide. As a result, we put ourselves in the ridiculous situation of driving the incredible machine just to burn off fuel. The relationship between consumption and exercise has become back to front.

DIETS DON'T WORK

You might see a flaw in this comparison between burning fuel in your car and burning fuel from your body.

When your car runs out of fuel, it stops running. But when your body runs out of fuel, it starts to draw on the reserves of fat, and that is exactly what you are aiming to achieve, right?

So, you drain your body's fuel and start eating into your fat reserves. But your body is crying out for fuel. When you stop exercising, you have to resist the temptation to eat; otherwise you will just replace what you have disposed of. It will take willpower, making you feel deprived and miserable. You might be able to keep this up for a while—you have probably been through similar periods of self-denial in the past—but all you are doing is dieting. And diets don't work.

Diets are short-term efforts to create an unnatural imbalance between intake and disposal and will usually result in short-term weight loss while you follow them. However, when you come off them, the weight piles back on, as you haven't fixed the cause of the original problem. In fact, they usually result in long-term weight gain. You put yourself through misery and deprivation and end up worse off than when you started. The good news is that the happy outcome you seek can come naturally and without willpower, provided you follow Nature's Guide as other animals do automatically.

WHY DO YOU EAT?

You might think this is one of those silly questions I talked about before. Obviously, you would die of starvation if you didn't eat. But when you sit down to eat, do you think to yourself, "I must eat this food to prevent myself from starving to death?"

I imagine starvation is, in fact, the last thing on your mind before a meal. How many of us actually know what starvation feels like? There was an occasion in my life when I was seriously concerned that I might die of thirst, but I don't think a day has passed when I haven't been fortunate enough to have something to eat.

If I tapped you on the shoulder as you sat down to your evening meal and asked why you were about to eat the food in front of you, wouldn't the more likely reply be that it's what you always do at this time of day?

Say I asked you the same question as you were buying a snack in the middle of the afternoon. Perhaps that would be habit and routine, too, or perhaps you had been compelled by the aroma of cooking or because you regard snacking as a source of enjoyment.

Boredom and restlessness are other common reasons for eating. They are also common reasons for smoking. You have been there: sitting at a desk trying to finish a piece of work that is becoming a drag. It's taking longer than you expected, and you are losing confidence in finishing it satisfactorily; you want some relief, so you reach for the cookies, chips, or a chocolate bar.

But when you have finished and you return to work, the problem is still there. The snack has not removed it. Let's face it—it was absurd to think it would.

So, the question is not that silly after all: you eat for all sorts of reasons, many of which are not hunger. Compare that to the rest of the animal kingdom. Animals do the opposite. They are driven to eat purely by hunger. The squirrel knew to stop eating nuts and start storing them. It had eaten enough to keep itself functioning and knew that because it was no longer hungry.

REVERSING THE CYCLE

Your relationship with exercise is affected by your relationship with food. If you overeat and try to exercise to burn off the excess calories, exercise becomes a chore and you will not be able to maintain it.

To avoid overeating, you need to rethink your relationship with food, so you treat the process as you would treat a car. That means eating nutritious foods that register on the hunger gauge and stopping when the gauge says "full."

Junk food acts against this rebalancing in two ways: first, it leaves you lacking in energy, gaining weight, and feeling despondent and unmotivated; second, it leads to addictions that create an illusion of false pleasures, which always seem more attractive than doing exercise.

Once you see through the illusions, you will begin to question your food choices. Nature intended for us to enjoy eating as part of our survival instinct. When you rediscover the foods that were intended for you, rather than junk, you will find that eating is actually more of a pleasure, not less. This will help you to enjoy exercise as a natural part of your life, not as a punishment that you feel obliged to put yourself through. However, do not feel compelled immediately to change what you eat just because you want to exercise. You will probably find it happens gradually and naturally in any case. And if you want some extra help with that, consult *Lose Weight Now* or *Good Sugar Bad Sugar.*

But something may still be holding you back—an inner suspicion that this cannot be as straightforward as I'm making it out to be. If you followed the second instruction— to open your mind—you should be starting to question your lifestyle choices and the beliefs behind them. Still, there may be a sense that there will be a price to pay. So, let's examine the thoughts that might be holding you back, starting with the most powerful emotion of all.

Chapter 9

FEAR

Fear is one of Nature's most powerful forces. It can drive us to run or fix us to the spot. The two faces of fear play a major role in the aversion to exercise. Let's examine your fears and help you dispel them.

You probably make a lot of excuses. People with an aversion to exercise tend to. They must make excuses because they know they are making the wrong choice and therefore feel the need to justify themselves.

Do any of these sound familiar?

"I'm just not feeling it today. I'll be up for it tomorrow."
"I haven't really got time for it right now."
"I've got a slight twinge that I don't want to aggravate."

And on and on it goes.

I had a friend called Mary who, when she was a young mother, used to look forward to her weekly gym class so much that she always made a big effort to put her baby to sleep in time for her to go. She would be so disappointed if the baby stayed up and made her miss class. That class was the highlight of her week.

Years later, I asked Mary if she was still going to the gym. She told me, rather sadly, that whereas she used to do everything in her power to make time for her classes, now she would let the clock tick until it was just too late for her to go. She would blame lack of time for missing out on the gym, but really, she was using time as an excuse to avoid going.

The telling thing was that in admitting this to me, she was clearly dejected that this had become her norm. "I don't understand why I do it," she said. "I love the gym and feel sad and angry with myself when I don't go. But something holds me back."

Two things were clear from this:

1. She was getting no pleasure at all from her decision not to exercise;

2. Some force she couldn't identify was preventing her from making what she knew was the right choice.

That force was fear.

You have been brainwashed into thinking that you derive some relief, comfort, or pleasure from avoiding exercise. So, despite the fact that you cannot actually put your finger on what that relief, comfort, or pleasure is, you fear being deprived of it.

At the same time, you are also aware of the detrimental effects you are inflicting on yourself by not exercising and worrying about the long-term consequences. You are caught in a tug-of-war between conflicting fears, and it makes you think contradictory and illogical thoughts:

"Every time I choose pleasure, I seem to end up feeling miserable."

SOMETHING THAT MAKES YOU MISERABLE
CANNOT BE A PLEASURE

Focus on that thought and get it clear in your mind.

IMAGINARY FEARS

We have a tendency to bury our fears. We don't like to admit we are afraid, especially when it relates to something as apparently insignificant as avoiding exercise. But this is a significant fear and not something to be ashamed of. Fear is an incredibly powerful force that controls much of our behavior.

It is also an instinct—part of our survival tool kit—the response that drives us to fight, flee, or freeze when faced with danger. Fear can be intellectual, too. For example, a horror film poses no real threat; there is no real danger, but the suggestion of danger is enough to trigger fear.

Humans imagine danger even where there is none. This is both an asset and a disadvantage. It helps us learn to cross the road safely. It also helps us behave in ways that safeguard our long-term future. For example, you might fear losing your job. That is a fear born out of reasoned conjecture. There may be no immediate danger of doing so, but you picture the consequences nevertheless, and that instills fear. So, you take steps to safeguard your job, even when there is no present threat of losing it.

This type of fear is helping you in this instance, but it can become an unhealthy burden. If that fear gets out of hand, it can make you permanently anxious when nothing is actually threatening you. Fear is designed to trigger an instant reaction and then to pass. We were not designed to remain in a long-term state of fear. But the human ability to project can make you permanently afraid of threats that don't exist AND NEVER WILL. Like the projected misery of what life might be like if you committed to regular exercise.

You know that your health will improve, yet you have been brainwashed into believing that some valuable aspect of life will be lost—as if all those times when you have chosen the couch over exercise have given you a pleasure that you couldn't bear to lose. However, instinctively you know that is not the case. In reality, you have absolutely nothing to fear from establishing a regular exercise routine. Moreover, incorporating exercise that you enjoy into your day gives you a *joie de vivre* that makes it easy to maintain.

You have been bombarded with so much false information that it's impossible to know what to believe until you test it out. As a result, you end up spending a lot of your life worrying about things that will never happen and not worrying about things that will.

Fear is the basis of your problem with exercise. It is the force that keeps you in the trap, afraid to take the simple steps that will lead to your escape. The trap is ingenious. When you tell yourself to do exercise, you wish you didn't have to. When you let yourself off, you wish you hadn't.

This is why you will never feel completely fulfilled until you conquer your aversion to exercise. When you are exercising, you wish you didn't have to. When you don't exercise, you wish you had.

THE FEAR OF FAILURE

The fear of failure can be a positive force. An actor waiting in the wings, a student going into an exam, an athlete on the blocks; fear of failure is the little voice in their head that forces them to focus, remember everything they have rehearsed and trained for, and leave nothing to chance. It can bring remarkable clarity of thought, judgment, and outstanding performance. However, when it comes to changing a behavioral trait like aversion to exercise the fear of failure can be a debilitating and self-fulfilling force.

The trap is similar to being in prison. There are no walls or bars; the prison is purely in your mind. But while you remain a slave to the brainwashing, you will experience the same psychological symptoms as an inmate in a physical jail.

If you have tried and failed to commit to regular exercise, you know that the failure leaves you feeling more firmly trapped than you did before your attempt. It's like that moment in a film when a prisoner is thrown into a cell and the first thing they do is run to the door and tug at the handle. This confirms their predicament: they really are locked in.

Trying and failing to overcome your aversion to exercise reinforces the belief that you are trapped in a prison from which there is no escape. This can be hugely dispiriting and enough to put you off trying again. You tell yourself that the best way to avoid the misery of failure is to avoid trying in the first place. Plus, as long as you never try to escape, you will always be able to preserve the belief that escape is possible. This twisted logic keeps you well and truly trapped.

Millions of people worldwide are trapped in this way— intelligent, otherwise rational people who tell themselves that the best way to avoid the misery of failure is not to try. What they don't realize is that the person who tugs at the prison door and finds it firmly locked is simply using the wrong method of escape.

You have already broken this cycle because you have chosen to try to escape. That is why you are reading this book. Easyway is the key. Tugging at the door handle is what people do on the willpower method. And the stronger willed they are, the longer and harder they will pull. This is why it's often strong-willed people who find it hardest to escape.

The fear of failure is illogical because the thing you are fearing has already happened. You are already in the trap. You have already failed. Every time you avoid exercise, you experience a feeling of failure, so using the fear of failure as an excuse not to try makes no sense.

This fear of failure is based on an illusion and unlike the actor's or the athlete's, which compels them to action, it compels you to inaction.

IF YOU SUCCUMB TO THE FEAR OF FAILURE, YOU ARE GUARANTEED TO SUFFER THE VERY THING YOU FEAR

There is another fear that can also keep you in the trap.

THE FEAR OF SUCCESS

There is a tendency for some ex-prisoners to re-offend within a very short time of being released. You might assume that these must be habitual criminals who know no better, but research has found that, in fact, many of them re-offend for no other reason than that they want to get caught. They actually *want* to go back inside.

Prison life is no picnic, but when it's the life you are used to, it can seem easier than the alternative. Life on the outside is unfamiliar and unnerving. You don't feel equipped to handle it. You are drawn back to the "security" of the prison.

Addicts have a similar psychology. They become afraid that life without their "crutch" will feel alien and disconcerting. They worry they won't be able to enjoy it or cope with its stresses and that they will be condemned to a life of insecurity, sacrifice, and deprivation.

When you have been brainwashed into believing that choosing to avoid exercise brings you relief, comfort, and pleasure, it's only natural to fear that choosing to do exercise will be no fun. This fear is just as powerful as the fear of failure. Although you are well aware that you do not feel happy when you avoid exercise, you may still have come to regard that choice as a symbol of your freedom to choose, indicating that you are a free spirit who doesn't slavishly stick to a given routine.

OK, so ask yourself:

Do I feel in control?
Does my avoidance of exercise feel like a free choice?
Am I really having fun not exercising?

Be honest with yourself, and then be absolutely clear: you will lose nothing of any value in your life by exercising. You will only make wonderful gains. You will feel more in control, freer, and have more fun because you really will be exercising freedom of choice.

This is what you will achieve: life without the slavery of being in the trap. It is not to be feared; it is something to look forward to with excitement. If you stay in the trap, you will feel that sense of failure for the rest of your life. This is NOT the life you were born for. You DO have a choice.

WIN THE TUG-OF-WAR

The trap makes you your own jailer. That is both its fiendish ingenuity and its fatal flaw. The panic feeling that makes you afraid to even try to overcome your aversion to exercise is caused by avoiding exercise. One of the greatest benefits you will receive is never to suffer that fear again.

The tug-of-war is a conflict between two fears: the fear of what your aversion to exercise is doing to you and the fear of committing to exercise and the unpleasant consequences that you associate with it. One of these fears is valid because it's based on fact; the other is invalid because it's based on illusions. Fortunately, the tug-of-war is easy to win because both fears are caused by the same thing: aversion to exercise.

START ENJOYING EXERCISE AND
BOTH FEARS DISAPPEAR

It would be great if I could transport you forward into your mind and body to the time when you finish reading this book and understand Easyway completely. You would think, "Wow! Will I really feel this good?" Fear will have been replaced by elation, the feeling of failure by optimism, low self-esteem by confidence, and apathy by dynamism. Your physical and mental health will be improved by these psychological transformations as well as by the actual exercise itself. You will look and feel fitter and you will enjoy both a newfound energy and the ability to truly relax.

People who rely on willpower to change some aspect of their lives always struggle because they feel that they are making a sacrifice. Get this absolutely clear in your mind:

YOU ARE NOT GIVING ANYTHING UP

You are getting rid of something from your life that makes you miserable and replacing it with something that makes you genuinely happy.

When you started this book, part of you believed that avoiding exercise was your relief, your comfort, your friend, and your guilty pleasure. It is essential that you recognize that this is an illusion brought about by brainwashing. In reality, the force that makes you avoid exercise is your worst enemy and, far from making you happy, it's driving you deeper and deeper into misery. You instinctively know this, so open your mind and follow your instincts.

REMOVE ALL DOUBTS

Think about all the wonderful things you will gain by starting to enjoy exercise. As well as the obvious benefits to your physical health and looks, think of the enormous self-respect you will gain and the relief of not having to make phony excuses.

There is only one way to remove the desire to avoid exercise:

START TO ENJOY EXERCISE!

As soon as you can see that there is nothing to fear, that you are not giving up anything or depriving yourself in any way, the transformation becomes easy.

So far, I've given you five instructions to put you in the right frame of mind to enable this book to help you overcome your aversion to exercise:

1. Follow all the instructions.

2. Open your mind.

3. Begin with a feeling of excitement.

4. Ignore any advice that goes against Nature's Guide.

5. Question your present tastes and eating habits.

If you are struggling with any of these instructions, go back and re-read the relevant chapters. It's essential that you don't just follow the instructions but that you also understand the reasoning behind them.

Making your transformation easy requires you to remove the fears that force you into inactivity: the fear of success and the fear of failure. You must be 100 percent certain about your desire to make this change.

SIXTH INSTRUCTION: NEVER DOUBT YOUR DECISION TO CHANGE.

As you continue through this book, you will be challenged to see things in a new way. This may cause you some doubts. It's fine to question what I say, as that will help reinforce the logic and truth behind it. But if you find yourself doubting your decision, remind yourself why you picked up this book in the first place and think about all the wonderful gains you stand to make when you achieve your goal.

Now, if you're absolutely sure about your desire to change but not so sure about your ability to do so, that is probably because you are not yet convinced that it's possible to succeed without willpower. It's time we dispelled this particular myth once and for all.

Chapter 10

WILLPOWER

IN THIS CHAPTER

• *SIDESTEP THE CONFLICT* • *WHY THE WILLPOWER METHOD
DOES NOT WORK* • *DO YOU REALLY THINK YOU ARE
WEAK-WILLED?* • *CROSSING THE LINE* • *BEWARE THE DIE-HARDS*

Human beings have achieved some incredible feats thanks to their willpower. The determination to overcome adversity is a remarkable *trait. However, using willpower to try to overcome your aversion to exercise will only make the problem worse.*

I have stressed all along that the change you want to make needs to happen easily. There should be no sacrifice, no feeling of deprivation, no suffering. Otherwise, you will be miserable and the change will not last. The transformation you are choosing to make is wonderful and will bring multiple benefits. You are making marvelous positive gains and losing absolutely nothing. What's more, with Easyway you won't even need willpower. Rejoice!

You may be thinking, "If it's so easy, why do so many people find it incredibly hard?" The answer is very simple: they are going about it the wrong way. The problem with other methods is that they involve suffering and misery. What is the point of even attempting a major change in your life if it does not make you happy?

Changing your attitude toward exercise is easy, yet even the simplest task can be made virtually impossible if you go about it the wrong way. Consider the simple act of opening a door. Push on the handle and it swings open with minimal effort. But if you have ever encountered a door with no handle and pushed on the wrong side by mistake, where the hinges are, you will know that it puts up quite a fight. The door might budge slightly, but it won't swing open. You would need a tremendous amount of effort and force to open it far enough to walk through.

Of course, you don't keep pushing on the wrong side, you change your method, push on the correct side, and the door opens effortlessly.

SIDESTEP THE CONFLICT

Your aversion to exercise will not be conquered by willpower. There is a general belief that exercise should be hard if you want to get anything out of it and that it requires effort and discipline to stick to it. This belief has been put in our minds by brainwashing. As we have lost touch with Nature's Guide and exercise has ceased to be an integral and automatic part of our lives, we have come to regard it as a chore.

The myth that exercise is hard is reinforced by the fact that most people use willpower to overcome their aversion to it. Because of the brainwashing, the temptation not to exercise can be strong, so there is a constant mental tug-of-war—a conflict of wills. Your rational brain knows you should exercise because it improves your physical and mental health, appearance, and self-esteem. But your brainwashed mind sends you into a panic at the thought of being deprived of those "couch slouch" temptations. Remember, those temptations are illusory. The pleasure you think you are choosing is false. It never leaves you feeling happy, whereas exercising does.

The easy way to resolve this mental tug-of-war is not to engage in it.. It's the brainwashing that you need to conquer. Once you do that by changing your mindset, one side of the tug-of-war disappears, as all your will is focused in the same direction, there is no conflict of will, and therefore no need for willpower. Does it take willpower to cross the road? Obviously not. But if you try to cross that road with your legs tied together, not only will you find it very difficult but you will also need to use considerable willpower.

WHY THE WILLPOWER METHOD DOES NOT WORK

Anyone who tries to conquer their aversion to exercise with the willpower method is fighting a losing battle. You focus on all the reasons for buckling down to regular exercise and hope your willpower is strong enough to keep going until the temptation to give up fades away.

This seems logical, but the problem is that you still feel you are making a sacrifice. This makes you miserable. It also makes you think you deserve a reward. And what do you do when you need a little reward? Let yourself off exercise. Very soon, you are back in the vicious circle and feeling even more miserable than before you made the attempt.

THE WILLPOWER METHOD MAKES A BAD SITUATION WORSE

The willpower method requires you to draw on your self-discipline to overcome the temptation to opt for what appears to be the easy option.

While the will to resist this temptation is winning, the will to succumb to it suffers and makes you feel deprived and miserable. Sooner or later, the balance shifts and temptation wins. Now, the will to resist temptation has been vanquished and you feel miserable because you have failed. You are miserable when you are exercising and miserable when you are not. You are fighting a battle that you simply cannot win.

Easyway resolves this conflict simply by removing one side of the tug-of-war, so there is nothing tempting you to avoid exercise and no sense of sacrifice. Unlike the willpower method, Easyway does not require you to draw on self-discipline; it takes away the temptation altogether.

SOME PEOPLE DO SUCCEED THROUGH WILLPOWER

There are some people who do manage to keep exercising through sheer willpower, but do they ever actually break free from the feeling that they are making a sacrifice?

DO YOU REALLY THINK YOU ARE WEAK-WILLED?

People often attribute their failure to quit smoking or drinking to a lack of willpower. Drug addicts are often branded as weak-willed as if that were the cause of their condition. But the reason people become addicts is not because they are weak-willed. It's because they started taking a highly addictive drug and persevered with it despite the huge costs to their well-being. Such behavior implies a strong will, not a weak one. The people who come to our clinics do not tend to be weak-willed or stupid. They are often highly intelligent, strong-willed characters who can't understand why they have failed to solve their problem for themselves.

If you think a lack of willpower is why you have been unable to overcome your aversion to exercise until now, you have not yet understood the nature of the trap you are in.

The fact is that everyone has an incredibly strong will at their disposal, and the strongest-willed people often find it hardest to quit on the willpower method. Why? Because they refuse to open their mind and accept that they have been brainwashed and are not in control. They cling to the illusion that they are making a sacrifice. They are stubborn. The more you struggle to get out of the trap, the more tightly ensnared you become.

TRYING AND FAILING IS MORE LIKELY TO BE A SIGN OF A STRONG WILL THAN A WEAK ONE

If you have assumed that lack of willpower is the cause of your problem with exercise, ask yourself whether you are weak-willed in other ways. Perhaps you are a smoker or a drinker, and you regard these conditions as further evidence of being weak-willed. There are many commonalities between all addictions, but none is a lack of willpower. In fact, addicts tend to be strong-willed.

What all addictions have in common is that they are mental traps created by misconceptions and illusions. When it comes to the issue at hand, one of the most damaging misconceptions is that exercising requires willpower. When you have been brainwashed into believing that doing something is going to be difficult and unpleasant, it becomes a self-fulfilling prophecy and you find excuses not to even try.

You know that exercise is good for your mind and body. You also know that you feel great after doing it and that you feel weak-willed and guilty when you avoid it. Yet you keep finding excuses for doing just that. This is not the behavior of a weak-willed person. It takes a strong will to persist in doing something that goes against all your instincts.

If you tried to open a door by pushing on the hinges and, despite being advised to push on the other side, you continued to push on the wrong side, I would call you willful, not weak-willed. The prisoner who re-offends soon after being released from prison is not weak-willed. They are displaying a strong will to get back inside.

There are plenty of high achievers who are hooked on alcohol, nicotine, or other drugs. How can the same person have the incredible willpower to get to the top of their profession yet be weak-willed when it comes to their addiction? It doesn't add up.

Are you really weak-willed? I'm sure you can find plenty of evidence to show that you are strong-willed. How do you react when people tell you to get more exercise? Don't you feel a strong urge to do the opposite? Wouldn't you describe that as willful?

When very strong-willed people try to change their addictive behavior by using willpower, they tend to find it harder than weaker-willed people because when the door fails to open, they don't give up and try another method—they force themselves to keep pushing on the hinges until they can push no more.

When people try to achieve a change in their lifestyle by using the willpower method, they never reach the finishing line. They remain vulnerable to relapsing into their old ways because they continue to believe that they have given something up, they will always feel deprived. And the more strong-willed they are, the more intense the feeling of deprivation will be. If you take away two children's toys, which one will scream loudest and longest, the weak-willed child or the strong-willed one? On the willpower method, you find yourself in a self-imposed tantrum. The hope is that if you endure the misery of the tantrum for long enough, the feeling of deprivation will go away. With Easyway, you remove the feeling of deprivation right from the start and therefore remove the need for willpower.

CROSSING THE LINE

When you quit with this method, there is a finishing line, and you don't have to wait to cross it. You do so as soon as you remove the brainwashing, the illusions, and the fears that cause you to avoid exercise. That is when you free yourself from the trap. You need to understand that you will not reach that point by forcing yourself to suffer.

We have helped tens of millions of people transform their lives, and we know first-hand that they do not respond well to the hard-line approach that the willpower method involves. Rather than helping, it actually impedes you because:

1. It reinforces the myth that achieving your objective is hard and therefore increases your fears.

2. It creates a feeling of deprivation, which you will seek to alleviate by doing the very thing that you want to stop doing.

You have probably already tried and failed to resolve your aversion to exercise using willpower. If so, you will know that it puts you off trying again because you don't want to repeat the unpleasant experience and may even have formed the belief that your problem is impossible to solve.

People on the willpower method often report a sense of relief when they first give in to their temptation to stop exercising. It's important to recognize that this relief is simply a temporary end to their self-inflicted suffering. It doesn't make them happy. No one celebrates their failure. On the contrary, they become furious with themselves and feel impotent and miserable.

It's important not to confuse pleasure with the relief of ending pain, particularly when that pain is self-inflicted. It's a great relief to take off tight shoes, but you wouldn't put them on just for the "pleasure" of taking them off!

BEWARE THE DIEHARDS

You probably know someone who is using willpower to stick to an exercise regime. Perhaps you admire their resolve and wish you could do the same. Don't! Remember what you have learned about the willpower method and see things as they really are.

Die-hards who try to change an aspect of their lifestyle by using the willpower method can have a disruptive effect on your own desire to change. They either boast about the sacrifices they are making or they moan about them. Either way, they reinforce the false belief that change necessarily involves sacrifice. Get it clearly into your mind:

THERE IS NO SACRIFICE

It's very important you understand that you are not giving anything up. As soon as you can see this, you will win the tug-of-war because your opponent will be powerless. Without the tug-of-war, there is no need for willpower. Take away the fear and there is nothing to tug against. It's easy.

People using willpower are forever waiting for the day when they can stop struggling, but with Easyway there is no struggle and nothing to wait for. As soon as you achieve the right frame of mind, you resolve the conflict of wills and remove the temptation to avoid exercise.

It's a fantastic thrill the moment you are free from your struggle. If you have followed all the instructions and understood everything, you should already be feeling a sense of anticipation and excitement. You have already taken a major step toward solving your exercise problem.

You will soon be in control and understand that nothing can prevent you from realizing your goal.

There is just one more possible factor that could be holding you back from feeling that you are regaining control. People who try to change and fail again and again put it down to something beyond willpower—a flaw in their character. If you have understood and accepted that your aversion to exercise, as I explained earlier, works in the same way as addiction, then you might also fear that it's part of your genetic make-up, a trait commonly referred to as an "addictive personality."

In the next chapter, we will examine the theory of the addictive personality and show you why this, like willpower, is not the source of your problem.

Chapter 11

WHAT IF I HAVE AN ADDICTIVE PERSONALITY?

You can be fooled into believing you can never overcome your problem with exercise because that is the type of person you are. The truth is, anyone can overcome an aversion to exercise and it has nothing to do with your personality.

We have established that your problem with exercise works in the same way as drug addiction and has nothing to do with a lack of willpower. There is a widespread assumption that it's incredibly difficult to beat an addiction and that it requires huge amounts of willpower. Easyway disproves both these assumptions: addiction is easy to cure provided you use the right method, and willpower is certainly not the way to succeed.

Even so, many addicts find it hard to believe that they can be completely cured.

ARE YOU THE PROBLEM OR THE VICTIM?

When you understand the way the trap works, you can see why an addict might think that way. Addicts make excuses, but they don't lay the blame on anyone else: not the big businesses peddling addictive poisons, not the role models who convinced them it was cool, not their peers or parents who unwittingly contributed to the brainwashing. Addicts blame something in themselves.

We don't like to think that our lifestyle choices are being determined by external forces, so when we keep making bad choices, we assume that the problem lies with us. When you keep ducking exercise, do you blame other people? Of course not.

You might brand yourself as weak-willed, lazy, helpless, or just unfortunately doomed to be unfit. Whatever criticisms you use, you assume that you are the problem.

An important part of taking control of your exercise problem is first accepting that the problem does not lie within you—you are the victim. Like millions of other people, you have been brainwashed, exploited, conned, and misled.

You should understand by now that the pattern of determination, sacrifice, reward, and relapse only occurs when you follow the wrong method. Relying on willpower creates a feeling of sacrifice and deprivation, so when you begin to think you are getting somewhere, it's natural to want to reward yourself.

When your brainwashed mind believes that the best reward you can give yourself is "just the one" —be that a drink or a cigarette or a break from exercise then you soon find yourself back where you started.

THE ADDICTIVE PERSONALITY THEORY

Blaming a lack of willpower for your problem is one thing. The addictive personality theory goes a huge step further in giving you an excuse to remain permanently in the trap.

It is based on the assumption that some people have a genetic predisposition to becoming addicted. No matter how hard they try, there is something in the way they are made that makes them addicts. It could be cigarettes, it could be heroin, it could be anything but exercise. They will inevitably get hooked on something, and once they are, they can't become free again. Their personality keeps them trapped.

Unfortunately, this hypothesis is subscribed to by certain scientists and, more importantly, perpetuated by the fellowship commonly known as Alcoholics or Narcotics Anonymous. Let me be very clear, I have no wish to denigrate this fellowship that many addicts swear by and credit with enabling them to abstain from alcohol and other addictive substances. I personally know numerous people, some of them close friends, who say they would be dead were it not for the fellowship and its twelve steps method, and I believe them. It therefore pains me to criticize it in any way. But criticize it I must, as it is perhaps the most influential proponent of the addictive personality theory, which prevents addicts from becoming mentally free. At its core is the myth that there is no cure for addiction—"once an addict, always an addict"—and that the problem is caused by some inescapable flaw in one's genetic makeup or personality. It states that addiction is an incurable disease and that the best one can hope for is a "satisfactory" life by remaining permanently "in recovery'" but never completely recovered. This is why its disciples are encouraged to continue attending meetings for the rest of their lives and to start each meeting by stating: "I am an addict," even if they haven't touched the addictive substance for decades!

If you are looking for an excuse to stay in the trap, this is perfect. Rather than having to tell yourself, "I know I should exercise this evening, but I'm going to duck it because I'm a hopeless, weak-willed jellyfish," you can tell yourself, "I really want to exercise this evening, but something in my genetic makeup is stopping me." You're not blaming anyone else, but you're also not really blaming yourself.

Many addicts pounce on the addictive personality theory for this very reason. The safety of the prison and the fear of quitting overrides their desire to become free and this gives them the excuse to stop trying. This is defeatist and miserable, but if you're in the exercise trap, it appeals to you because:

- You believe ducking exercise gives you pleasure or comfort.

- You think the alternative will involve suffering.

- You are afraid of failure.

So what do you believe? If you are still under these illusions, there is something you have not understood, and you need to re-read the relevant chapters about fear and brainwashing. It is essential that you understand and have no doubt whatsoever that:

- Ducking exercise gives you no genuine pleasure or comfort whatsoever; it merely gives you a temporary and illusory relief.

- Becoming free is easy when there is no conflict of wills.

- While you remain in the trap, you have already failed and a life free from the aversion to exercise will leave you feeling amazingly good compared to how you feel now.

COMMON TRAITS

The addictive personality theory came about because scientists studying addiction noticed certain similarities between addicts that seemed to suggest a common trait. These were:

- Continuing to crave their fix years after quitting.

- Getting hooked on multiple addictions.

- Getting hooked much more severely than other drug users.

- Sharing personality traits with other addicts.

We can dismiss the relevance of these apparent consistencies one by one.

CONTINUED CRAVING

Addiction is largely a mental condition, not a physical one. If you quit without removing the belief that your "fix" gives you pleasure or comfort, you will tend to continue feeling deprived, and you will have to continue to fight temptation.

MULTIPLE ADDICTIONS

It is common for people with an aversion to exercise also to be drinkers, smokers, over-eaters, and, in many cases, all of these. They are all caused by the same thing, but it's not the personality of the addict. It's the misguided belief that the thing they are addicted to gives them a genuine pleasure or comfort.

MORE SEVERE ADDICTION

Why do some people fall deeper into the trap than others? For example, why did I smoke 100 cigarettes a day when most people seemed to manage on 20? This does indeed point to a difference between us, but there are numerous differences between people that can explain why one person's behavior differs from another's in this context. None of them has anything to do with personality or genetics.

The way we behave is governed by all sorts of influences. As we grow up, we are all subjected to different conditions and role models: parents; teachers; friends; things we read, watch and listen to; places we go, people we meet, etc. These are all part of the brainwashing, and they will all have a bearing on how quickly we descend into the trap. People with time and money on their hands tend to fall into the trap faster because there are fewer obstacles holding them back.

If you believe that you get pleasure or comfort from avoiding exercise, and each time you do, you feel that little boost caused by the partial relief from the craving for that moment of indulgence, then your belief will increase, your desire will increase, and your determination to keep ducking exercise will increase.

It is the belief that your alternatives to exercise give you pleasure or comfort and your ability to indulge in them more often and in greater quantities that speeds up your descent into the trap.

SHARED PERSONALITY TRAITS

If, until this point, you have resisted the idea that your problem works in the same way as an addiction, you may change your mind when you think about the common shared behaviors:

Repeatedly trying and failing to quit.

Feeling inadequate, guilty, and ashamed.

Lying to yourself and others.

Making excuses.

Feeling low regularly.

Do you recognize these in yourself? They are commonly reported among people struggling to maintain regular exercise. Does this mean they all share the same personality defect? Of course not. They are symptoms of the problem, not the cause of it.

Addicts share them because that is what the trap does to you. It controls you and makes you conceal your condition out of shame, leaving you feeling weak, frustrated, and miserable.

You may feel that you and other people in your predicament are a different breed from everyone else. You may well feel more comfortable in their company as a result. Beware of the temptation to believe that your shared behaviors are evidence of a shared personality flaw that has doomed you all to have an aversion to exercise.

People tend to seek the company of those with the same problems, not because they are more interesting, free-spirited, or fun, but because they feel more comfortable around people who won't challenge them or make them confront their problem. You all know that you are doing something illogical and self-destructive. If you are surrounded by other people doing the same thing, you don't feel quite so weak. These destructive feelings of weakness, stupidity, and hopelessness are a terrible reality. You will recognize them after you give in to the temptation to avoid exercise. They are the chief cause of your misery and the chief reason you are reading this book.

The good news is that once you are free, you won't just be spared all the unhealthy effects of avoiding exercise, you will also be liberated from its terrible impact on your mental well-being.

DEBUNKING THE THEORY

The addictive personality theory is just that—a theory or hypothesis, and it does not stand up to scrutiny.

It is based on genetics. It assumes there is a gene that predisposes some people to addiction. If that were the case, it would follow that there would be a fairly consistent proportion of the world's population who are addicts.

But this is not the case. Take smoking, for example, the addiction about which the most data have been gathered over time. We know that in the 1940s, over 80 percent of the UK adult male population were smokers. We also know that today that figure is under 14 percent. A similar trend is evident throughout most of the West. So are we to conclude that the proportion of people with addictive-personality genes has fallen by a whopping 66 percent in just over half a century?

While the percentage of smokers in Europe and North America has plummeted, the percentage in Asia has soared. So what has happened there? Have all the people with addictive personalities migrated to Asia?

Cases of obesity and diabetes are soaring, but no one is putting this down to the addictive personality theory. It is quite rightly being blamed on the increased amount of junk food on the market and the barrage of brainwashing from advertisers encouraging people to consume it.

Your struggle with exercise is not caused by an addictive personality. If you think you have an addictive personality, it's simply because you are hooked and have found it impossible to escape so far. This is the trick that the trap plays on you. It makes you believe that you can't get by without your false pleasures because there is some weakness in your character or genes. Addiction maintains its grip on you by distorting your perceptions.

The addictive personality theory reinforces the belief that escape is out of your hands and that you are condemned to a life of frustration and misery. This is a myth created by the illusion that the alternatives to exercise give you pleasure or comfort and that resisting them will involve a sacrifice. See through the illusions, deconstruct the myths, and escape will be easy.

The frustration and disappointment of your aversion to exercise will soon be put behind you as you continue to absorb this book. Once you can see the situation in its true light, you will wonder how you were ever conned. Like millions of people around the world, you have been the victim of an ingenious trap. Recognize the trap for what it is, dismiss any idea of a flaw in your personality or genetic makeup, and you will be ready to walk free.

Chapter 12

SEEING THINGS AS THEY REALLY ARE

You have passed the halfway point in this book, and you are well on your way to establishing the new mindset you need to overcome your aversion to exercise. Let's take stock of what we have learned so far and consider some practical steps to help you plan your escape.

I don't expect you to grasp everything set out in this book immediately, but it is important that you follow all the instructions and understand and accept the reasoning behind them.

Now is a good time to recap and ensure you are absolutely clear on everything I have told you so far. If there is anything you are unsure about, please go back and reread the relevant chapter. Remember, the method works like the combination that unlocks a safe and you risk failing to apply it successfully if you don't understand each step as you go along.

PERSONALITY AND WILLPOWER

We have established two very important facts about your exercise problem:

1. It has nothing to do with a lack of willpower.

2. It is not caused by any weakness or flaw in your character but is the result of misconceptions. These are being removed by this book.

When you choose to skip exercise in favor of something that seems easier, it may feel like a failure of willpower on your part, but that is not the case. In reality, you are suffering from a conflict of wills caused by misunderstanding. You know you want to exercise, you know it will make you feel good both physically and mentally, and yet you still choose to avoid it because you have the wrong mindset.

FEAR

Two basic fears lie at the root of the problem. The fear that trying to exercise more will be a grueling experience and ultimately end in failure. The fear that even if you do succeed, you'll have to spend the rest of your life using willpower to resist the temptation to give up on it. Both these fears are illusions caused by brainwashing, which Easyway is already removing.

As long as you are controlled by these fears, you will not be able to overcome your aversion to exercise. Remove them, and you will find it easy.

THE INCREDIBLE MACHINE

We have recognized that the human body is an incredible machine, equipped with all the tools and gauges required not only to survive but to enjoy life and maintain a healthy balance between the fuel we consume and the fuel we burn off. By ignoring those gauges (our senses), we lose that balance and suffer the consequences in the way we look, feel, and perform.

How way we look, feel, and perform is the main driver behind our desire to do regular exercise. In order to look the way we want, to feel relaxed and free from guilt and self-loathing, and to perform with energy and clarity of mind, we know we need to exercise. We don't just know this because we have read it in books or been taught it at school. We know it instinctively. Instinct drives us to exercise. Remember those children rushing around all day without a care in the world before the brainwashing got to them.

We know it intellectually too, because there is a vast amount of information in the media about the benefits of exercise for the body and mind. But this intellectual knowledge is undercut by a conflicting force—the brainwashing we are subjected to from the day we are born. Our instinct to exercise is undermined by the belief that there are always better, more enjoyable, and less arduous ways to spend our time.

This illusion is what holds you back. Remove the brainwashing, follow your instincts, and exercise will feel like the most natural and enjoyable thing on earth.

FUELING UP AND BURNING OFF

We have established that there is a direct connection between what you eat and your inclination to exercise. By eating the right foods—those that are easiest to digest and quickly give us the nutrients and energy our body needs—we can strike a natural balance between intake and output, maintain an ideal weight, and shake off the lethargy that results from a constant consumption of junk.

This is because hunger, the gauge that tells us when to eat and when to stop, responds to the nutritional content of what we consume, not the volume. When we eat junk, the hunger gauge hardly responds because there is very little nutrition, so we tend to stuff ourselves, become sluggish, lose energy, and feel disinclined to exercise.

You don't have to stop eating junk altogether because the incredible machine, your body, can tolerate a certain amount. But if you consume mainly junk, not only will you have weight problems but you will also seriously undermine your chances of overcoming your aversion to exercise.

THE TRAP

We have also established that your problem is not your fault. You have been deceived by a cunning web of brainwashing and illusions into thinking you are applying free will when in fact you are not in control of your choices. You have been caught in a fiendish trap.

The trap cleverly cons you into believing the opposite of the truth. For example, it convinces you that avoiding exercise will make you happier when you know from experience that the opposite is true. This tug-of-war between what you know instinctively and what your brainwashed mind tells you deepens your confusion and inner conflict, which in turn makes you less able to escape the trap. This is exactly how addiction works. The problem is in your mind.

Without changing your mindset, you will never conquer your aversion to exercise permanently. The great news is that when you do change your mindset, breaking free is easy and, most importantly, so is staying free.

SEE THROUGH THE ILLUSIONS

If you are clear on all these points, then you should be starting to see through the illusions that keep you in the trap. For example, the illusion that because human beings today are much more sophisticated than our ancestors, we don't need to be as physically active.

The human body has evolved very little over the last million years, and the design that helped our ancient ancestors survive and become the dominant species on earth is the same design that made you. So, let's look at some more of the myths and illusions that make you averse to exercise.

1. Exercise is mindless

Some people regard exercise as a mindless pursuit—it's OK for athletes and bodybuilders but not for cerebral human beings. It's a form of intellectual snobbery that provides an excuse for physical indolence. In fact, as I write this book, I can't resist the urge to go for a quick ride on my bicycle from time to time, followed ideally by a quick cold shower to reinvigorate not just my body but also my mind. I do my best thinking and writing immediately after exercise. The body is relaxed and the mind is sharpened by an increased clarity of thought.

People who exercise daily find they really miss it when they stop. Once they have experienced the physical and mental benefits daily, they are loath to forego that feel-good sensation.

2. Exercise hurts

Contrary to the "no pain, no gain" mantra, exercise is not supposed to hurt. If it does, stop. Pain is a sign that you are doing something harmful to yourself. That defeats the purpose of exercise.

But it is worth noting that much of the pain we associate with exercise is imaginary. We expect it to be painful, so we feel pain when we do it. The mind is very powerful when it comes to creating false perceptions out of expectations. The good news is that you can easily train your brain to think the opposite, especially when the opposite is true.

Next time you do an exercise that you think is painful, ask yourself, "Is this really hurting? Is this really pain?" If you are expecting pain and you feel the need to breathe deeply or a mild burning sensation in your muscles when you are exercising, you may interpret that as pain. In fact, if you take the trouble to analyze it at the time, you will recognize that it's nothing of the sort and can even train yourself to enjoy it.

3. Exercise is boring

Perhaps you had a PE teacher at school who made you do repetitive and seemingly pointless exercises. Perhaps you have spent time in a gym repeatedly lifting weights or running on a treadmill. If you found that boring, then you may naturally associate all exercise with tedium.

Exercise can be repetitive, but it does not have to be boring. You can make it as fun and stimulating as you like. Playing sports is great exercise, great fun, and it's virtually impossible to be bored while doing so. Cycling, swimming, dancing, walking, and numerous other forms of exercise are among our most popular forms of recreation, not because they involve physical exertion but because they are enjoyable in themselves, and you feel great afterward.

Boredom is a state of mind that sets in when you are unstimulated. Exercise has the opposite effect. It triggers hormones that make you feel stimulated and fulfilled.

4. Exercise takes up too much time

Who says how long you have to spend exercising? You can exercise for as long or as little as you like. Even short bursts will produce noticeable benefits, as I find on bike rides. One of the great things about exercise is that the more you do it, the more you want to do it because the more you genuinely enjoy it. It's the opposite of the vicious cycle that you were stuck in when you started this book.

If you think you don't have time for exercise, think about what you do instead when you goof off. Don't you usually do nothing much? It's OK to relax and do nothing sometimes, but it's hardly an antidote to boredom or a recipe for an interesting or exciting life. And the problem is that the more time you spend doing nothing, the harder it becomes to do anything else.

5. The alternatives to exercise are more relaxing

This is a very common misconception. True relaxation is a combination of physical and mental calm. It's easy to achieve physical calm by sitting on the sofa watching TV, but mental calm is not so straightforward. You can sit doing nothing for hours, but your mind is unlikely to be relaxed. And if you are feeling guilty about not exercising, your mind will never settle.

If you want to feel truly relaxed, exercise first. In fact, mental calmness will set in while you are exercising. Just ask people who like to go running. They will tell you it takes them to a restful place in their mind that they can only ever find through exercising.

6. The alternatives to exercise are more fun

We have established that some of our favorite forms of recreation involve vigorous exercise. What could be more fun? A party? Meeting friends? Watching TV? Sure, these can all be great fun, but none provide the hormonal stimulation and afterglow of satisfaction and joy that come with exercise.

As long as you believe that when you avoid exercise, you are choosing pleasure over pain or fun over tedium, you will remain in the trap. See through the illusions and recognize the truth: the human body is not only physically but also mentally stimulated by exercise. If you think your life lacks stimulation and fun, exercise more.

RESET YOUR ASSUMPTIONS

Get it clearly into your mind, your avoidance of exercise is not a matter of free choice. It's the result of brainwashing. Your choices are being controlled by illusions. After all, if you could choose freely, you would be doing more exercise. That's why you're reading this book.

As you unravel the illusions and begin to see the truth about exercise and what it does for you—and the truth about the things you do instead of exercise and what they do for you—you will shatter these illusions, get back in touch with your natural instincts, and become free to start enjoying exercise again, just as you did as a child.

You now need to replace the illusions preventing you from exercising with accurate perceptions. Be clear that exercise is not a form of torture you have to endure to improve your health. It is a completely natural and enjoyable activity in its own right, with its own built-in reward system. It is a source of genuine pleasure, as natural as breathing. Denying yourself the freedom to enjoy exercising is as unnatural as keeping an animal in a cage.

The best guide to when to exercise and when to stop is not an artificial regime imposed on you by a book on fitness or by an instructor, it is your own natural instincts. As you recognize the power of your instincts, you will become more attuned to what they are telling you and you will be more inclined to acknowledge the vital signals they send you.

WIN THE TUG-OF-WAR

The fears that keep you in the trap are all the result of illusions. As you see through the illusions, you will dispel the fears. You will see that treating yourself to regular exercise will make life more enjoyable.

Once you overcome the fear of becoming free—the fear of success—you remove any conflict of wills, and winning the tug-of-war becomes easy. Without any reason or desire to avoid exercise, you will quickly lose the fear that you don't have what it takes to overcome your problem—the fear of failure. You will actually begin to seek out opportunities to exercise. You will not be able to resist it.

Then you will be free of the two major fears that keep you in the trap. Instead, you will establish a virtuous cycle of exercise, satisfaction, energy, and confidence, which you can enjoy for the rest of your life.

ENJOY THE EFFORT

You will be amazed by the transformation. Simply by questioning some deep-seated assumptions, you will establish a new mindset that gives you a whole new, more positive outlook. You will be healthier, happier, more energetic, more confident, and more in control.

This is an incredible feeling. I wish I could transport you into that state right now, but don't worry, you will experience that transformation very soon. You may even be starting to feel it already.

Without the brainwashing and misconceptions that created your aversion to exercise, you will start to enjoy it in a way you never thought possible. Rather than seeing the effort and exertion as a pain, a chore, or a bore, you will enjoy it in itself and welcome it as a natural sign that you are doing yourself good.

You will recognize the difference between the false pleasures that have distracted you from exercise and the genuine pleasure of exercise itself—a pleasure that is not followed by a low but by a lasting high.

The amount of effort you put in is entirely up to you. Your incredible machine will tell you when you have had enough. Listen to it. It's the best guide.

Whichever forms of exercise you choose, be sure to apply yourself to them enthusiastically and with joy. That might seem like a tall order given your past experiences. Remember, those attempts were driven by a sense of obligation and entailed willpower. They weren't driven by enthusiasm and so did not involve elation.

WHY BE ELATED?

Imagine you haven't been feeling well for a while. You're tired all the time, feeling aches and pains, breathless after walking up a staircase or running for the bus, feeling sluggish and generally out of sorts. Your sleep hasn't been great, you trudge around at work feeling uninspired and listless, and you avoid doing almost anything that involves effort. So, you visit your doctor who does some tests. They book you an appointment to revisit them in a week to get the results.

As each day passes, you begin to worry about what might be wrong with you. As you become increasingly anxious, you hope for the best but begin to fear the worst. What is it? Is it treatable? What if it isn't? Will it get better? Will it get worse? What if it never gets better? What if it's something dreadful, untreatable, and life-threatening? You try not to think about it, but that makes you obsess about it even more each day and you feel more and more stressed.

You start noticing and appreciating simple things: the sun shining, birds singing, leaves blowing on the branches of the trees in the wind, the joyful sound of children playing, the comfortable home you live in, and the friends and family you haven't seen for a long time. Your mind turns toward things you used to enjoy but for some reason stopped doing, places you wished you had been but never got around to visiting, things you wished you had done.

Eventually, the appointment with the doctor comes around. As you knock on the door, a feeling of dread floods through your body. You walk in, take a seat, and hope for the best. The doctor looks concerned. It's not good news. You're told that as things stand, your situation is bad and is likely to get progressively worse. Apparently, you can expect more unpleasant physical and mental symptoms such as a severe increase in the aches and pains, more weight gain, mood swings, depression, and eventually much worse. Your life will become increasingly difficult and you should prepare yourself for a painful, unpleasant, and undignified death. You ask how long you've got. The doctor tells you he can't say. Not knowing adds to your feeling of panic.

You wish with every fiber of your being that this is an awful nightmare. But it isn't. This is real. Panic turns to terror.

"Doctor, please, is there nothing that can be done?"

"Actually," the doctor says, "there is something."

"What? There is hope? I'll do anything, pay anything, go anywhere, if I can be cured! If the treatment is successful, is my prognosis good?" you ask.

"Excellent," the doctor says.

"Wow! Is it expensive?" you ask.

"No, not at all. In fact, it won't cost you a penny."

Your mind is racing. Hope has suddenly returned. "Are there side effects or pain?"

"The treatment is drug-free and painless, but there are some quite considerable side effects," replies the doctor.

Your heart sinks again, but side effects are better than no hope and a slow and painful death.

The doctor continues, "You can expect the following side effects: improved mood, a greater sense of happiness, less anxiety, less stress, more energy, greater vitality, better sex ... " You interrupt, incredulous and confused, "What? These are the side effects?"

"I haven't finished," the doctor says. "You can expect a better, fitter body shape, less bloating, fewer aches and pains, better sleep, and weight loss."

Your jaw drops. This is extraordinary. You've gone from the depths of despair to the pinnacle of hope. You can't wait to start the treatment.

How would you feel about undertaking the treatment? Would you be reluctant and resistant to it? Would you follow the treatment with a begrudging lack of enthusiasm? Of course not. You'd look forward to starting it as soon as possible. You'd undertake as much of the treatment as you could possibly manage. And you'd do so with enthusiasm. And you would smile every step of the way. Wouldn't you?

As you've no doubt already realized, the scenario described is your own. And you have the treatment plan, the key to your escape right now.

Bear in mind, I'm not saying that to look at it this way you'll immediately be able to kid yourself into doing what's needed for you to get into shape. This is not fiction. Now is the time for you to start getting better and embrace a whole new quality of life—with a smile on your face!

It doesn't matter how out of shape you might be, you can benefit from exercise immediately.

Whatever your current physical or mental condition, something very special is about to occur in your life. You are embarking on that amazing transformation described by that doctor, and it will be dramatic and more thrilling than you can imagine. You will notice the physical improvements very quickly and you don't have to wait a second to enjoy the psychological benefits. Exercising is so great for our mental health that it's proven to be far more effective at combating depression, anxiety, and stress than anti-depressants or anything else a doctor might prescribe. Enjoy your freedom right from the start.

PRACTICAL STEPS

It's simple and easy to take immediate action to counter our increasingly sedentary lifestyles.

Introducing some brisk walks of twenty to thirty minutes is virtually effortless even if you're currently very unfit, and every minute beyond the twentieth makes a huge difference. From around the twentieth minute, your body is revved up and the blood flow is greatly increased, which helps kick-start your metabolism and lift your mood. You'll soon be enjoying it so that you'll be doing thirty minutes or more without any effort at all.

Sports are a fantastic option and there are plenty to choose from whether you fancy playing tennis, softball, volleyball, etc., or team sports like soccer or basketball. Sports have two main advantages. The first is that once you find a sport that you enjoy, playing it is completely effortless. You focus on having fun and don't even notice that it's exercise. The second is that it usually involves social interaction, which is also a great thing in itself.

There are lots of fitness apps and on-line guides for a range of abilities to choose from if you like the idea of those, as well as apps to help with yoga, Pilates, etc. The danger of these is that they can start to feel like a chore, like going on a diet, if you're not careful. Do not think that you have to stick to any regime imposed on you by anyone else. Your body will tell you when to stop. Start getting more in touch with it and follow what it and your instincts are telling you. If it starts to hurt, stop. There are many social options too, such as classes at sports centers and gyms. Choose something you will enjoy rather than something you feel you "have to do." Whichever you choose, once you start exercising again, you'll love it. It's all about making yourself feel great.

Cast off any sense of doom and gloom and feel genuinely excited and enthused about how much better you're feeling.

Cycling is also marvelous. If you live within cycling distance of work, I strongly recommend you commute by bike if possible. If you don't already have one and have the space to keep one out of the rain, get one and start using it for journeys you would otherwise have made by public transport or car. It will save you a fortune in transportation costs, and in cities it will save time too. One of the other great advantages is that you always know exactly how long a journey will take, as traffic doesn't affect you. Don't worry if you are not initially confident cycling on the road. Urban planners have finally woken up to the huge merits of cycling in cities and have made it much safer and easier by introducing bike lanes, bike rentals, etc. You'll get used to it in no time and be amazed at how practical it is. You can pick up used bikes cheaply on-line and will get your money back many times over in no time at all. Don't be put off by the weather. Once you get into cycling and have proper clothing, it soon becomes second nature, virtually regardless of the weather.

If cycling on the road isn't for you, then an exercise bike is an excellent option if you have space. It can be worth buying one— again you can pick up a used one cheaply—rather than signing up for a gym membership. Fitting in twenty to thirty minutes of exercise at home is much more time and cost-efficient than driving to the gym, and makes adding it to a busy schedule far easier. It also has the advantage of being weather-proof. Finally, exercise bikes also allow you simultaneously to enjoy entertainment in your home. You can watch your favorite TV shows or films in twenty- to thirty-minute installments while peddling away.

Walking is fabulous exercise and can be enough to make a significant difference in itself. Instead of going on autopilot when you walk, focus on how you feel and pay attention to how your body moves, the rhythm of your footsteps and the air on your skin. This is known as walking mindfully and you can easily work it into your daily routine and the fact that it's making you feel physically and mentally better adds to the other elements of enjoyment it will bring.

If you have to drive, rather than walk or cycle, to work, appointments, light shopping, sports events, or shows, always try to park your car farther away than you might ordinarily. Finding a space close to an attraction or event can be both expensive and frustrating. Driving around trying to find a space is so much more stressful than making sure you're not in a rush, parking farther away and enjoying a walk.

It's extraordinary how much easier and less pressured life becomes when you make simple changes such as this. So many of us feel the desperate need to park as close as possible to where we're going without realizing that it's adding to our stress levels, and there's a much easier option. Also, if you're worried about the environment, it has the added bonus of reducing your emissions.

Experiment getting on or off the bus/train/subway a stop or more from where you would normally. You'll find yourself increasingly enthusiastic about it the more you do it.

I previously mentioned walking mindfully, but there's no reason why you shouldn't use your walks for entertainment and learning purposes too.

Books: these days, most books are also available as an audiobook (my own included), so there's never been an easier time to enjoy their content while getting out and about.

Podcasts: with so many "free to listen" podcasts available, you can catch up with your favorite self-help, comedy, sports, or current affairs programs while on the move.

Music: whichever music platform you love, you can enjoy walking to a playlist of your own or let the platform algorithm do it based on your preferences or listen to your favorite artists' albums.

BEWARE OF INJURY

Injury can stop you in your tracks, so always do a few stretches before any exercise that might strain your body, and take things easy to begin with. If you do pull a muscle or injure yourself, you don't have to stop exercising, you just need to change the exercise to avoid aggravating it.

Being ill can obviously impede you. You shouldn't exercise if you've come down with the flu or some other temporary illness that drains your energy and makes you feel lousy. Look forward to exercising again as soon as you're better. The more exercise you do, the fitter and healthier you become, and the less susceptible to illnesses you will be.

As well as the more energetic twenty- to thirty-minute exercise ideas mentioned, it's also important that you move your body, even for a few moments every so often. Sitting or laying down for long periods, other than while sleeping, isn't good for us and can cause serious illnesses. The main reason so many people have deep vein thrombosis issues on long-haul flights has nothing to do with flying and is solely related to remaining completely immobile for lengthy periods. It's also a risk for people who are hospitalized and not able to move.

If your work involves sitting down for long periods, here are some ways to keep healthily active:

- Consider not reacting to social media/messenger notifications without standing up for a stretch or walking to the water cooler to read them. You'll check notifications less frequently, waiting for a few to build up (which is great for focus and reducing smart-phone use). You'll also stand and stretch more often when you do check them. It's a good balance.

- If you are a professional driver, make sure that you take a walking break to stretch your legs as often as possible.

- Have some standing or walking meetings if possible. They tend to be shorter than seated meetings, far more productive, and allow you to move.

- Stand up when you're on the phone, and work standing up for periods. Just standing, rather than sitting, is exercise in itself.

- If you work in a large office, use the bathrooms farther away from your desk. If that involves using the stairs, even better.

- Set an alarm for every fifty to sixty minutes to remind you to move.

The same "not sitting for lengthy periods" advice applies to those lazy evenings watching TV:

- Get up for a stretch or walk up and down the stairs between episodes of your favorite show.

- If you have more than one bathroom and stairs, only use the one that's a flight of stairs away. It's not Mount Everest!

- Doing chores that involve movement that you normally avoid, knowing that your partner or house mates will do them, will make you healthier and also more popular.

Whichever forms of brisk exercise you choose, and whichever of the "move your body more often" strategies you adopt, you can start doing them without any great effort and after a very short time of repeating them, they will become automatic and completely effortless.

This book will remove your aversion to exercise and kick-start your enjoyment of it. This change in mindset is often accompanied by a reassessment of other aspects of your lifestyle and a desire to make additional positive changes. If that happens to you, it's important that you don't use the willpower method to try to achieve them. If you do, you might undermine your ability to apply Easyway to the problem we are currently resolving. As you know, Easyway offers help with many issues which also improve fitness, health, and well-being. On pages 221–224, you will find a list of these. So, while this book is all you need to succeed in attaining your exercise goals, if you want to make other changes, then please take a look at the range of Easyway programs and books available.

Don't delay your new exercise plans until you read them though. They will help you once your freedom to exercise is achieved. Together, the books have helped more than 50 million people just like you to change their lives for the better.

Chapter 13

BE KIND TO YOURSELF

IN THIS CHAPTER

•*AN EXERCISE-FRIENDLY DIET* •*THE JUNK MARGIN* •*A REGULAR SLEEP PATTERN* •*EXERCISE FOR PLEASURE* •*THINK POSITIVELY*

You are ready to reverse the vicious cycle and create a positive mindset. This can be fueled by a powerful combination of lifestyle choices around diet, sleep, and exercise, all of which complement each other.

I have explained how exercise is a natural part of human behavior, something our ancestors did without a second thought. As our civilization has evolved and we have developed ways of acquiring food that doesn't require us to forage, we have come to regard exercise as an artificial activity conceived by other humans to help us stay fit and healthy.

It's important to change this mindset. Rather than seeing it as a chore that you need to do when you want to lose weight or get stronger, embrace it enthusiastically as an enjoyable part of a well-rounded healthy lifestyle. It can then become part of a package of natural processes that together amount to being kind to yourself.

Along with exercise, that package includes diet, sleep, and mental health, and they all feed off each other. Try to create the right conditions for exercise. That means establishing a positive state of mind, which is helped immensely by eating and sleeping well. The better you eat, the better you sleep, the better you feel, and the more able and inclined you are to exercise.

We have focused a lot so far on mindset: removing the brainwashing, myths and illusions, the fear and negativity, and replacing them with a clearer view of the truth and a positive approach to overcoming your problem. Now, it will help you to start thinking about your diet and sleep to create the all-round conditions best suited to exercise.

AN EXERCISE-FRIENDLY DIET

Do you ever ask yourself why you eat? It may seem a strange question. Obviously, if you didn't eat you would starve to death. But that is not what you think every time you eat, is it? "I must eat or else I will starve to death."

In fact, the most common drivers for eating are:

Routine
Temptation
Boredom
Restlessness
Sociability

It's great to eat according to a routine, provided that routine is in sync with your body clock. The actual reason you eat is to give your body the fuel it needs to fulfill its many functions. In this respect, it is very much like a car. Do you fuel your car by putting in the same amount at the same time every day? Of course not. If you did, there would be times when the fuel tank overflowed, spilling gas everywhere.

To help us know when the car needs fuel, manufacturers provide us with a fuel gauge. Your body also has a fuel gauge: hunger. Hunger is the signal that your body is running low on nutrients and needs to refuel. For an exercise-friendly diet, try to pay attention to your natural fuel gauge, just as you would pay attention to the gauge in your car.

People tend to eat more or less the same quantity of food every day around the same time because that is their accustomed routine, and that's fine if it fits in with the needs of their body. But do you sometimes eat because you are craving sugar, and a cake or bar of chocolate looks tempting? Or because you are bored or restless? Or because it's a social occasion and there is lots of food and everyone else is tucking in? When you eat for these reasons, you are likely to overfill the tank.

Unlike the car's fuel tank, the excess has nowhere to go and is converted into fat and excess weight. This becomes a source of stress and anxiety, which can have a detrimental effect on your sleep, your state of mind and your attitude to exercise.

Remember, the hunger gauge indicates the level of vital nutrients in your body, not the quantity of food that you have put in your stomach. When the level is low, you feel hungry. Eat foods that are low in nutrients, and you will go on feeling hungry. In order to get the nutrients you need and top up the gauge, you have to eat more, creating more waste and building up more fat.

The process of digesting what you eat itself consumes a lot of energy if you are eating foods which the body finds hard to break down. Unlike exercise, which leaves you feeling great, this drains you, making you feel tired even when you haven't exerted yourself. This is why you feel lethargic after eating a load of junk. Your attitude to exercise is directly related to your levels of energy. If you are not feeling energetic, it's only natural that you will feel averse to exercise. The body is sending you signals to rest. It can't send you signals to exercise at the same time. As well as giving you a negative attitude to exercise, lethargy and tiredness caused by a poor diet also make it harder to sleep. In fact, it makes it harder to do anything at all!

When you eat in response to hunger, you stop when the tank is full. Chances are you will still eat according to a regular routine because that is how your body clock works. But the types and quantity of food you eat will vary according to how much you burn off.

When you eat nutritious foods—particularly fruit, vegetables, nuts, and seeds—the hunger gauge quickly registers full with very little waste. That's because these foods are easy to digest, and the nutrients quickly go where they are needed. The food tastes great and leaves you feeling revitalized and brimming with energy. It doesn't overflow as fat. You don't have to bother yourself with special diets or vigorous exercise to burn off fat. All you have to concern yourself with is your intake of fuel, i.e. what you eat.

PLEASE RE-READ THE PARAGRAPH ABOVE AND MAKE SURE YOU HAVE UNDERSTOOD IT! IT IS VERY IMPORTANT!

Eat slowly to allow for the time lag while your body absorbs the nutrients it needs, and this registers on the fuel gauge. With fruit, vegetables, and nuts, you don't have to wait as long as with meat, which takes a very long time to digest.

So, the recipe for an exercise-friendly diet is to eat nutritious foods when you're hungry and stop when you're not. Savor the flavor and notice the gauge responding. You will find that you enjoy your meals far more and you will feel fantastic. Remember, if you stop eating before you feel completely full, you'll find the inclination to eat more invariably disappears. The tendency to overeat will then disappear.

You don't have to give up any foods. Just try to eat a lot of fruits, vegetables, nuts, and seeds. Our bodies can digest a wide variety of foods. It's just that some take more time and energy than others, and we have to eat more of them to get the nutrients we need, which leads to obesity and lethargy.

For an exercise-friendly diet, try to eat mainly nutritious foods. You will quickly start to feel the benefits in terms of energy, peace of mind, and sleep. Furthermore, as you reconnect your senses with your eating, you will start to recognize that nutritious foods are actually the most pleasurable, and your desire to consume junk will diminish.

This is a natural process that happens gradually. Unlike dieting, which forces an abrupt change on your body and leaves you feeling deprived, focusing on nutritious foods (fresh vegetables, fruit, nuts, and seeds), without forbidding yourself any particular food, means eating and drinking remain a pleasure and you will find that the more you focus on healthy foods, the less you will want to eat unhealthily.

A REGULAR SLEEP PATTERN

How often do you wake up before your alarm goes off? Even say, when you change your alarm to 4 am because you have to catch a flight, it's very common to wake up before it sounds. Your body just seems to know, doesn't it?

The body clock is incredibly sophisticated and the above is an example of how it manages our physical and mental processes without us being conscious of the fact. Think of your body clock as a multitude of different clocks, each regulating different parts of the body. It works best when all those clocks are in sync.

So, while your mental clock might wake you up at 4.00 am to catch your flight, the rest of your body is not in sync, and you feel tired as you drag yourself out of bed. As the body clock readjusts, that tiredness will catch up with you later in the day or even a day or two later.

For healthy sleep, keeping the body clock consistent and regular is important. That means getting into routines around when you go to bed, when you get up, when you work, when you unwind, and when you exercise.

I mentioned earlier that when you eat should be dictated by hunger, not routine. That is absolutely true. But just as you build a routine for all the other activities in your life, hunger will align with your body clock, and you will find that you feel hungry at the same times every day.

You will notice that I said "when you go to bed" and "when you get up," not "when you sleep" and "when you wake." That is because the sleep-wake cycle is controlled by the body clock. All you can do is create the ideal conditions for sleep and ensure you can sleep when your body clock is ready.

By keeping to a regular routine, you will find this easy. Be prepared to make adjustments as you pay attention to your body's signals. Perhaps you are lying in bed for ages before falling asleep and could comfortably go to bed later. Nothing should be set in stone, but when you find a routine that works for you, try to stick to it as a general rule.

With your body clock in sync, you won't even have to think about it anymore. Sleep will come naturally, night after night, and you will find more energy for exercise when you are awake.

EXERCISE FOR PLEASURE

Thanks to the ingenuity of the incredible machine, exercise is also a major benefit to sleep. Research has shown that exercise helps both with getting to sleep and enhancing the quality of the sleep you get. It is particularly beneficial for deep sleep.

Hormones released during exercise also help to regulate your mood and control the sleep-wake cycle. The production of these hormones through exercise helps to alleviate stress and anxiety, putting you in a more relaxed mental state, which naturally aids sleep.

And, of course, the effect of exercise on weight is a further benefit to sleep. People who maintain regular exercise as part of their lifestyle are far less prone to obesity, which is a major cause of sleep disorders. Having said that, weight loss should not be your motivation for exercise. Exercising, like eating, is a pleasure. To prove this point, the body actually produces chemicals that make us feel good after exercise.

Exercising to lose weight is like driving your car just to burn off fuel. The motivation is flawed. Feeling overweight causes a negative mindset, and the exercise we do to try to shed pounds tends to feel more like a punishment—the "no pain, no gain" mentality.

Do you really want to punish yourself? When you eat an exercise-friendly diet, you don't need to because your intake takes care of your weight. It is all in balance. It's when you ignore Nature's Guide and overdo the junk that things go wrong.

SEVENTH INSTRUCTION: EXERCISE FOR PLEASURE.

There are two important reasons for this. The first is that the pursuit of pleasure is what we are trying to achieve by curing your aversion to exercise. The second is that choosing a form of exercise that you enjoy will mean you stick with it, and it will become an effortless part of your lifestyle.

This doesn't happen when you exercise to lose weight. You push yourself to burn off the pounds, and once you get down to your target weight, you reward yourself by giving up the exercise and returning to your previous lifestyle. Surprise surprise, the weight piles back on.

"Exercise for pleasure" is not a difficult instruction to follow. There are innumerable choices when it comes to exercise, and they can all be fun, provided you are doing them with the right frame of mind.

THINK POSITIVELY

The amount of exercise you take and the time of day you choose to take it are entirely up to you. There are no set rules.

The more you enjoy your exercise, the more you will want to do it. The more you do it, the more fuel you will burn off. The more fuel you burn off, the hungrier you will feel, and the more you will enjoy the nutritious food that will encourage you to exercise more.

It's a wonderful cycle, and it works in any quantity. Do little exercise and you won't feel so hungry. You will eat smaller portions, still get the nutrients you need and maintain a healthy body.

Your body will tell you when and how much to exercise. Some people are capable of running marathons, while others are better suited to a walk or some light indoor exercises. Most people find exercising first thing in the morning stimulating as it kick-starts their circulation and puts them in a good mood that can last the whole day, but exercising in the evening is also fine—it's whatever works best for you.

Establishing a complementary relationship between exercise, diet, and sleep will help you achieve everything you want from exercise. That is the beauty of the incredible machine: it is designed to make you feel good when you do things that are good for it. You will get the most benefit not by putting yourself through pain but by being kind to yourself. That doesn't mean ducking exercise; it means embracing it as a vital and enjoyable part of your newly balanced lifestyle.

As you establish this harmonious balance, you will naturally feel more positive, energetic, optimistic, and happier. That is what happens when you follow Nature's Guide.

Isn't it great?! Instead of approaching exercise with a feeling of doom and gloom, you can look forward to it with excitement, knowing that every time you do it, you will feel better and better both in body and mind.

Chapter 14

REVERSING THE BRAINWASHING

IN THIS CHAPTER
•*EXERCISE YOUR SENSES*
•*YOU DON'T HAVE TO GIVE UP ANYTHING* •*AVOID SUBSTITUTES* •*KILLING THE MONSTERS*

As you rebuild your naturally positive mindset toward exercise and its complementary package of sleep and diet, it's also important to remove any influences that can disrupt that balance and undermine your escape from the trap.

The willpower method involves fighting the temptation to indulge in something you believe is a pleasure or crutch. With Easyway, there is no need to fight because you remove that temptation altogether.

People find it hard to change their behaviors because they believe in two myths:

1. It means sacrificing something that they truly enjoy or depend on.

2. The process is difficult and involves suffering.

The first myth can be dispelled by focusing on the belief in the pleasure or crutch and realizing that it's an illusion.

Having done that, the second myth can be dispelled simply by using the Easyway method. Without the illusion of pleasure, the process is not only easy but also enjoyable.

When you take a conscious approach to your lifestyle choices and can see through the brainwashing, the illusion of pleasure or benefit of any kind dissolves. When you understand how the process works, you realize that it's only the nature of the trap you're in that has prevented you from solving your problem. By seeing through the illusions and understanding that avoiding exercise gives you no genuine pleasure or relief, you remove the brainwashing. The reason you have repeatedly avoided exercise until now is because you have been the victim of an addictive process that we are dissecting in this book, and you will soon be free.

By stopping to question the way you spend your time instead of exercising and what you eat and drink, you give your natural instincts the power to help you follow Nature's Guide. This is the enlightened approach. You reconnect with your senses, and by paying heed to what your incredible machine is telling you, you unravel the brainwashing and start seeing things as they really are.

At the same time, you reap the rewards of your new lifestyle choice. You feel fitter and healthier from exercising and the nutritious foods you eat and gain all the wonderful, restorative benefits of a good night's sleep.

Most importantly, you regain control of your life. You may convince yourself that by avoiding exercise, you are asserting control by making your own decision, but deep down, you sense you are being controlled because you would prefer to be making a different choice. This creates confusion and self-loathing—two stressful mental states that are hugely damaging. When you escape the trap and remove your aversion to exercise, you take back control. There will be clarity in your decisions, your self-esteem will rise, and you will enjoy a profound sense of empowerment and liberation.

EXERCISE YOUR SENSES

When I talk about reconnecting with your senses, you may be wondering what I mean exactly and how you should go about it. Perhaps you feel you are already connected. After all, you can probably feel, see, hear, taste, and smell. Your senses seem to be in working order.

That's great, but are you really paying attention to what they are telling you? We are so conditioned to believe what we are told, rather than what we can sense for ourselves, that the connection with our senses has become weak. You can strengthen the connection in the same way as you strengthen any other facet of the incredible machine—through practice.

Walking is a great time to exercise both your body and your senses. As you walk, pay attention to the world around you.

Notice the sounds, the smells, the colors, and the shapes. Feel the ground under your feet and the air on your hands and face.

You can exercise your senses on any walk. It doesn't have to be somewhere serene or picturesque, like the countryside or the beach. A walk while shopping or out running errands offers the same opportunities for connecting with your senses.

Most of us walk without paying attention to our surroundings. Often, we have our eyes on the pavement, lost in thought. Walking is very good for thinking. It helps you de-stress by giving you time and space to sort through your thoughts and develop plans and solutions. And that's fine. But remember that there's also great joy to be had from experiencing the world around you through your sensors: your eyes, your ears, your nose, your taste buds, and your skin. So, when you are walking, try keeping your head up and paying attention to everything around you. As well as enjoying the here and now, you will notice how your brain feels calmer and more alert at the same time and quicker to make connections between all the information it's taking in.

You will also remember more. Do you ever have that feeling when you are driving that you can't remember anything of the last five minutes at the wheel? You wonder how you avoided crashing because it feels like your mind was completely switched off. The human brain has the power to do this when performing familiar tasks. It can shut off conscious thought but still respond to the information coming in through the senses, like an autopilot.

The downside is that you are detached from the present and your life passes you by without you truly experiencing it.

We spend a lot of our time in this state, automatically performing familiar tasks. We pursue many behavioral patterns in the same state rather than paying attention to how they really make us feel.

It's very easy to change this. You just need to make a conscious decision to do so. Practice when you are walking, eating, socializing, or doing any of the other activities that you enjoy. Bring your senses to the party. Use them to get the most from the experience. And listen to the signals when they sound a warning.

Alternatively, tech now makes it possible for us to listen to books, podcasts, or our favorite music while we're walking. It can be truly relaxing to do so. Whether you walk mindfully or listen to your favorite playlist, walking will be fun and highly beneficial to your body and mind. You may enjoy it so much that you end up investing in some proper gear so you don't miss out on cold or rainy days.

YOU DON'T HAVE TO GIVE UP ANYTHING

Using your senses this way will enable you to distinguish between genuine pleasures and false pleasures.

Pay special attention to the things you tend to do instead of exercise and use your senses to examine them thoroughly. Ask yourself how you feel as you are doing them. "Is this making me feel relaxed?," "Does this taste good?," etc. You will quickly detect when something is not right, and you can then make any changes you want.

It's essential to understand that you are not giving up anything. I have made the point throughout this book that you don't need willpower to cure your aversion to exercise. In fact, relying on willpower is counterproductive. You only need willpower if you have a conflict of wills. For example, when you are doing some vigorous exercise, your muscles start to tire and your body sends a message to your brain to stop. You then have to use willpower to override that message if you are to carry on. That is willpower in action.

When you decide to change your lifestyle for the better, why would any part of you question that decision? That would only happen if you believed that you were making a sacrifice—giving up some sort of pleasure or crutch. In that case, you would need willpower in order to resist the temptation to relapse into your old ways.

If you are on the willpower method, you are laboring under the illusion that you are making a sacrifice, so there is a constant battle going on in your mind between the desire to keep at it and the desire to give up—the mental tug-of-war. Even if your willpower holds out for the rest of your life, as long as you continue to believe that you are making a sacrifice, you will always feel deprived.

Most people do not hold out. Their willpower eventually cracks, and they become more firmly imprisoned than before because they have now proven to themselves that escape is impossible.

As you identify the harmful aspects of your current lifestyle, take pleasure in the thought of banishing them from your life. You are not making sacrifices, you are clearing out rubbish and making space in your life for more of the good stuff. When you see that, you will find there is no conflict of wills, so you won't need willpower.

Be clear in your mind that the changes you are making are purely for the better. Anything that distracts you from the pleasure of exercise is your enemy, and the only reason you might think otherwise is because you have been brainwashed. You have already come a long way toward unraveling the brainwashing and should now understand how the addictive process cons you into thinking you need things that actually do you nothing but harm.

Avoid using the expression "I give up" when talking or thinking about any of the lifestyle changes that you want to make. Giving up implies a sacrifice. This is not a sacrifice, it's shaking off the bonds that have kept you trapped and unable to commit to regular exercise. That is a great feeling. It is freedom.

Chapter 15

TAKING BACK CONTROL

IN THIS CHAPTER
- *THREE STEPS TO FREEDOM* • *THE MOMENT OF REVELATION*
- *A NEW PLAN FOR EXERCISE* • *INITIAL RESISTANCE*

It's time to start rebuilding your lifestyle around choices that give you genuine pleasure. Fortunately, these choices are also the best for your health and happiness.

Some people skip straight to this part of the book without reading anything beforehand, hoping to find an instant fix. If that is you, sorry, but Easyway does not work like that.

Up to this point, the book has been preparing the ground for creating the ideal conditions for your new, positive approach to exercise. Without reading the whole book, you will not have laid the groundwork, and the plan we are going to look at in this chapter alone will not provide the solution. If you have skipped straight to this page, please go back to the start. That is all you need to do.

If you have read and understood everything up to this point and followed all the instructions, well done! You are fully prepared.

Exercise makes you feel good and is essential for health and happiness. When you find it difficult to commit to exercise, or just don't feel like it, or other distractions pull you away, the cause has nothing to do with how you were made or your personality. This is great news because it means you can do something about it. You don't have to go on suffering the cycle of lethargy, inactivity, and disappointment, nor the physical effects caused by a lack of exercise.

You should be clear about this now. Your aversion to exercise is not something you are permanently lumbered with, and while you may have felt helpless in the face of your inability to stick to regular exercise in the past, you are about to take back control. It's not about imposing a new regime on yourself, it's about learning how to enjoy achieving your goals.

We have already identified some of the lifestyle choices that may have been holding you back and preventing you from creating the ideal conditions for enjoying regular exercise. You may even have started to do something about changing them. If you have followed all the instructions, you will have kept an open mind to everything you have read so far, and you should be seeing things very differently. You will understand that things you used to regard as a pleasure or a comfort are actually part of a mental trap which has resulted in an aversion to exercise.

You now understand how the trap works and why you find yourself in it. You should be in no doubt that there is nothing to give up. On the contrary, you are losing absolutely nothing and only making marvelous, positive, life-changing gains.

If you have any doubts about the changes you are making, keep this point in mind and remember the sixth instruction: Never doubt your decision to change.

Other people may be skeptical. They may even tease you. Laugh it off. They are probably in the trap themselves and wish they could find a way out, as you are doing now. Remind yourself what you are achieving: you are freeing yourself from the harmful physical effects of lethargy that could develop into something critical at any time; you are freeing yourself from the mental fear of that outcome; you are freeing yourself from the feeling of slavery and frustration that comes with being trapped. By freeing yourself from these physical and mental impacts, you are giving yourself the freedom of health and happiness.

THREE STEPS TO FREEDOM

Ingenious though it is, the trap has one fatal flaw: you, the prisoner, hold the key. You are in charge of your own release. To escape, you just need three things to happen:

1.   You must recognize that you are in a trap.

2.   You must recognize that you hold the key.

3.   You must be shown how to use the key.

This is how Easyway works. Everything you have read so far is designed to help you see the trap you are in and recognize that you hold the key.

At the root of the trap is an addictive process. By understanding how this process works, you render it powerless and by creating the ideal conditions for regular exercise, you lay the ground for your escape.

The key is to unravel the brainwashing by questioning everything with an open mind and arriving at the truths behind the illusions and by reconnecting with your senses and your body's signals. Once you see through the illusions, you will never be fooled by them again.

The final step is to turn the key and walk free. We will look at that in more detail in the next chapter.

These are the three steps to taking back control of your life. By making different choices happily and of your own free will, you will enjoy a hugely enhanced quality of life and a marvelous feeling of empowerment and elation.

THE REVELATION

So, how do you know when you have fixed the problem? I've mentioned before that you never really become free with the willpower method because the brainwashing remains in your mind, always sowing seeds of doubt. With Easyway, you win the tug-of-war the moment you shatter the illusions and change your mindset. What does that feel like? It varies from one person to another. Some describe it as a "eureka" moment when everything clicks into place and the truth appears in sharp focus. Others are unaware of a particular moment and just sense that somehow their attitude has completely changed.

Look back at the illustration on page 57. Look at the three figures and remember what it felt like when you first realized that, despite clearly seeming to be different sizes, they are all in fact the same size. Also, look back at the GOOD/EVIL graphic below the figures. You now have the clarity to see the truth behind the illusions, and it's a power that you are about to use to change your life.

You don't need fireworks or fanfares to tell you when you have attained the right mindset. You just know. You see things differently. You notice things you didn't notice before. Confusion and helplessness have been replaced by clarity and confidence.

You can celebrate your triumph and get on with living your life the way you want to live it. Just as you will find other people questioning your new approach, you may experience moments of difficulty when some of the old feelings come back. This is perfectly natural, and there is no need to panic. It does not mean that you are still in the trap; it's just the old routine taking a little time to wear off. It won't last long and you don't have to wait for anything to happen. You can get on with enjoying your new life right from the start.

A NEW PLAN FOR EXERCISE

You may have started this book expecting practical advice on how to exercise in a way that you can sustain and enjoy. That is indeed what this book is all about. But it is not achieved by giving you an exercise program; it is achieved by preparing the ground—your mindset and lifestyle—to be receptive to any exercise program, routine, or way of living that you choose to adopt.

You can go about introducing exercise into your daily activities in many ways.

Think about what you have read and list as many as you can below.

If you are really excited by the idea of more vigorous exercise, go for it. Most gyms can provide help and advice on drawing up an exercise plan that is tailored to your needs. As you do so, keep the following tips in mind:

1. Be clear about what you are exercising for.

    Whether you want to train toward a specific target, such as a marathon or triathlon, or you simply want to feel fitter and more flexible, it helps to have your goal in mind. This will help you sustain your interest and enjoyment. Even vigorous, lung-bursting exercise is enjoyable when you have the right mindset and know that it is helping you to achieve your aims.

2. Tailor your exercise to your goals.

    Knowing what you are trying to achieve from exercise helps in arriving at a type, frequency, and level suited to you. The better your plan suits your objectives, the easier it is to maintain. This is important for two reasons: first, an exercise program that demands too much from you can cause injury, which defeats the object; second, if you find the exercise takes too much effort, you will cease to enjoy it and your motivation to continue will be undermined.

3. Make it enjoyable and sustainable.

    There is a tendency to exercise as an antidote to something else in your life that needs resolving, such as a weight problem caused by a bad diet or too much alcohol, and to rush into it headlong. This is not sustainable. It is far better to start slowly and build up. Such is the nature of the incredible machine that the more you exercise it, the more capable it becomes. Unlike a car, it doesn't wear out, it becomes stronger, provided you don't overdo it. So, take it easy to begin with and then challenge yourself more as you grow accustomed to it. This way, you will avoid injury, maintain your enjoyment, and continue to get satisfaction indefinitely.

4. Keep a diary of how you feel.

    Your capacity for exercise is not constant. It fluctuates according to many factors, such as biological changes, workload, relationships, diet, etc. A good example is the female menstrual cycle, during which hormone levels vary a great deal, affecting energy levels, susceptibility to injury, and other key factors. It is important to adapt your exercise to such varying conditions so you can ease off when appropriate.

INITIAL RESISTANCE

Even though you may already be looking forward to launching yourself into exercise with a new vigor, be prepared for anything that might undermine you. If you do find yourself struggling to muster the enthusiasm for exercise at any time, instead of telling yourself, "Here we go again! I'm losing my will," stay calm, remind yourself that you are making a major change to your whole lifestyle and there may be some resistance as you rid yourself of the harmful lifestyle choices that have been there for so long. Any change, even those obviously for the better, can take a little time to adjust to, like getting used to driving a new and better car or settling into a new and better job. These lingering pangs are simply your brain and body adjusting to the changes you are making and eliminating the last remnants of conditioning and brainwashing. Providing you respond to these in the correct way, they are nothing to worry about.

The odd pang you may get as you adjust to your new life when you make the decision to exercise rather than to do anything else, can be useful as a reminder of the wonderful gains you are making. The key is how to react to the pang. If you say to yourself, "Oh no! I've got to resist this temptation by using my willpower," you will feel deprived. If instead you say to yourself, "This is just my brain and body readjusting to my new life. Isn't it marvelous that I am not controlled by that pang anymore and can choose to exercise instead, take back control and enjoy my new-found freedom," you will be happy.

The pang may nag for a little while, but you can actually take pleasure from it by using that nagging feeling to create a mental image of a parasite inside you getting weaker and weaker, and you can enjoy starving it to death.

Keep this mental image ready at all times, and make sure you never respond to the pangs by feeling deprived and instead respond by thinking, "This what prevented me from exercising before but now I can enjoy exercise and very soon that little parasite will die I will never have to hear from it again." That way, these moments, instead of being an obstacle, can become times when you reinforce your joy at being free.

Be ruthless. Take pleasure in starving the parasite to death. As long as you are prepared, you will find it easy. You now have complete control over it. It's no longer destroying you; you are destroying it, and soon you will be free of it forever.

That way the pangs are no problem and usually disappear very quickly. After about three weeks, you may realize that they have gone completely. It's an exciting feeling.

When you realize you have been enjoying exercise without even thinking of bunking off, you can celebrate the pure joy of being free.

Keep it clearly in your mind that you are not making a sacrifice by exercising; that you can enjoy it while you are doing it and will feel great afterward; that whatever you would have done instead would have left you feeling dissatisfied, and that you will soon be doing it without a second thought. Above all, remember that you are making marvelous positive gains both physically and mentally and that you are losing absolutely nothing.

Any apprehension you might feel is just last-minute nerves, like a parachutist about to jump. You know that you have prepared everything perfectly and that the jump will feel exhilarating. You are the lucky fly on the wall of the pitcher plant that is being given the chance to fly away. Take it!

Remind yourself of all the things you stand to gain:

More energy
Better health
Greater contentment with your appearance
Better moods
Higher self-esteem
Less stress
Clearer thinking
Better performance
Better body shape
And, most importantly of all: greater happiness.

All of this is not just because you are exercising regularly but also because you have regained control of your life.

Chapter 16

BECOMING FREE

IN THIS CHAPTER

•*LOOKING FORWARD TO EXERCISE* •*CHOOSING YOUR MOMENT* • *WHAT IS THE BEST TIME TO CHANGE?*

You are now ready to make your move. You have all the knowledge and tools required to achieve the objective you desired when you began this book. It is now time for action.

The way you see yourself is a hugely important factor in your overall well-being and happiness—in fact, it is the most important factor. A person can have all the trappings of success, but if they are not content with the person they see in the mirror, they will not be happy.

That does not mean it is all about appearance. When I refer to the person in the mirror, I mean the way you perceive yourself entirely. Are you strong or weak, capable or incapable, resolute or flaky, kind or selfish...? When you have a problem like an aversion to exercise, you can quickly become very self-critical. "I'm so weak-willed," "I'm so flaky," "I'm hopeless," "I'm doomed to being a failure," "I hate my body," "I'll never be happy with the way I look."

This negativity adds to the problem, driving that vicious cycle that sends you in search of some sort of comfort or crutch. Because of the brainwashing, you seek comfort in the very things that create the cycle of misery: addictive substances and behaviors. One of the greatest benefits of reversing the cycle is that self-criticism turns to self-respect, self-loathing to self-love. You start to appreciate your body for the incredible machine that it is, and your confidence and self-worth grow.

This is very empowering. When you believe in yourself and your ability to take back control of your lifestyle choices, you begin to feel the incredible power we all have at our disposal. You were not born to be brainwashed, addicted, or consigned to a life of frustration, failure, and self-loathing. On the contrary, you were born to enjoy life to the full.

As you reverse the brainwashing, this truth begins to emerge. All the myths that you have labored under, which have kept you imprisoned and prevented you from fulfilling your desire to enjoy regular exercise, begin to melt away and a much clearer, more rational and positive reality takes their place.

The brainwashing and the illusions which resulted from it made you see yourself as a failure, powerless to overcome what seemed to be a weakness in your character. By now, you should be absolutely clear that your problem with exercise has nothing to do with your character but with the choices you have made in your life, which have clouded your view of reality and conned you into thinking there are more pleasurable things to do than the things that will make you truly happy.

When you were a child, if someone had asked you what sort of life you would like to lead when you grew up, would you have said "active" or "inactive?" Would you have chosen to be enslaved by addictions or free to make your own lifestyle choices? Would you have chosen a diet that carries the risk of weight problems, immobility, tooth decay, heart disease, and diabetes over one that gives you energy, health, fitness, and vitality? These are all choices we make in adult life, but the seed is sown in childhood by our parents and all the other influences in our lives. The good news is, you can change them and you can find it easy and enjoyable to do so.

When you can see that your aversion to exercise is not a flaw in your character but the result of a fiendish trick that has brainwashed you into seeing things in reverse and believing in a false reality, it becomes easy to change your approach and find the commitment that had eluded you.

When you can see yourself not as a hopeless failure with no willpower, doomed to a life of disappointment and frustration, but as an incredible natural phenomenon equipped with all the tools to survive and thrive, it becomes easy to change your self-image to one of a person making the most of your incredible powers and skills, and the natural inclination is to keep doing the things that genuinely make you feel good.

LOOKING FORWARD TO EXERCISE

When you establish harmony and balance between diet, sleep, exercise, and mindset, you set in motion a virtuous cycle that becomes self-powering. It does not matter where the circle begins; each stage drives the others. Regular exercise leads to better sleep, greater health, and vigor, and less stress and anxiety and thus, a greater inclination and capacity for exercise.

The virtuous circle of regular exercise

The vicious spiral of aversion to exercise

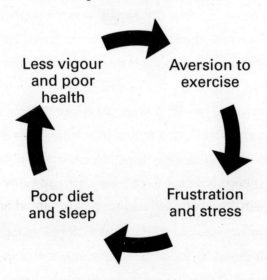

The virtuous circle of regular exercise

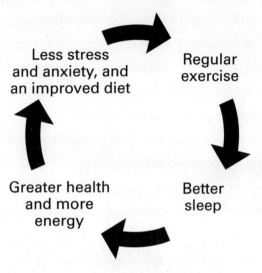

Your problem with committing to exercise has been a source of stress and anxiety in itself. You would no doubt begin to dread the moment when you promised yourself you would actually do some exercise, knowing that you would probably be lured away by temptations that would leave you feeling unfulfilled and yet seemed so hard to resist. When the moment came and you bailed out again, you were left feeling disappointed and frustrated with yourself, which added to your stress.

As you begin to apply your new lifestyle choices, you will attack the vicious circle of aversion to exercise at multiple points. You feel better about yourself. You reduce your exposure to stress and anxiety. You need less rest and enjoy better sleep. You build your health and vigor through a better diet, exercise, and rest, so you feel more inclined and ready to exercise.

This is the natural cycle that all creatures are designed to go through every day. It is the natural cycle that you were born to follow. It is effortless and self-powering. Once you get it turning again, it will run itself, provided you continue to follow your new routine.

You will be happy to do so because it is a wonderful routine that releases the hormones that make you feel good and motivated to do more. You will look back on the time when you feared that the change you needed to make would leave you feeling miserable about life and you will wonder what on earth you were thinking.

Now, you can look forward to exercise with the same joy that you would look forward to coming home to a loved one. Exercise, no matter how vigorous or gentle it may be, will become one of the highlights of your day, and the thought of it will fill you with joy and confidence, not the dread you used to feel.

You can look forward to exercise in this way right from the start. While it may take a little time to reverse the cycle fully, you will begin to notice improvements straight away. That is the sign that the method is working. The vicious cycle has disappeared, and the virtuous circle is purring into action.

Imagine how that will feel. Rather than dreading getting around to exercise each day, you can look forward to it with nothing but pleasure, knowing that the fear of a lifetime of inactivity is behind you and you never again have to worry about the effects of a lack of exercise on your body and mind.

It is a wonderful feeling. Until you restore the healthy cycle, you cannot fully gauge how heavily your exercise problem weighs down on you, both physically and mentally. It is a crushing pressure that increases over time and slowly squeezes the life out of you. It's an awful feeling, a constant worry at the back of your mind, and you try to bury your head in the sand and hope that one day it will resolve itself.

But bad lifestyle choices do not resolve themselves. On the contrary, they become increasingly destructive until you do something positive to change them. Only when you reverse the vicious cycle do you realize what a burden aversion to exercise really was. Its impact on sleep, diet, and mental health is highly destructive. Breaking free gives you a marvelous new lightness of spirit and feels like emerging from darkness into light.

CHOOSING YOUR MOMENT

So, you are ready to make your escape and now you just need to pick the right moment. The tendency is to choose an occasion that represents some kind of milestone, such as a birthday or New Year's Day.

I call them "meaningless days" because they have no particular bearing on your problem; they just provide a target date. You may consider them a line in the sand, but they can actually sabotage your bid for freedom.

New Year's Day is the most popular of all meaningless days, being a clear marker of the end of one period and the beginning of another. "New Year, new me!" You may be surprised to learn that people who choose midnight on New Year's Eve to make a major change happen to have the lowest success rate. I'll explain why.

The Christmas holidays are a time when people often eat and drink to excess, and by New Year's Eve, you are just about ready for a break. So, as the clock strikes midnight, you vow to embark on a new, healthy lifestyle. It may begin well, and after a few days, you may be feeling cleansed and good about yourself. But because you chose to quit on a day that has no direct relationship with how you are feeling about the problem you are trying to solve, you are unlikely to be in the right frame of mind and therefore will probably start to struggle.

Meaningless days encourage you to go through a damaging cycle of half-hearted attempts to quit, bringing on feelings of deprivation, followed by a sense of failure that reinforces the belief that change is probably beyond you. People with an aversion to exercise are always looking for excuses to put it off. Meaningless days also provide an excuse to say, "I will get down to it, just not today."

Having said that, please don't worry if reading this book happens to have coincided with one of those days. You are following Easyway, so you'll be in the right mindset anyway and if it happens to be your birthday or New Year's Day, this will not undermine you in the slightest.

Some people choose their annual holiday, thinking that they will be able to cope better away from the everyday stresses of work and home life and the usual temptations. This approach might work for a while, but it leaves a lingering doubt: "OK, I've coped so far, but what about when I go back to work?"

With Easyway, you remove your aversion to exercise first and then take the necessary action, so there is no need to avoid any situations that life presents. It is a great opportunity to prove to yourself from the start that, even at times when you feared you would find it hardest to apply yourself, you are still happy to be throwing yourself into exercise with a new *joie de vivre*.

SO WHEN IS THE BEST TIME TO START?

Let's go back to the door analogy. When you are stuck in the trap, trying to escape by willpower, it is like trying to open a door by pushing on the side where the hinges. If you had been pushing fruitlessly on the wrong side of the door and then discovered you could open it easily by pushing on the other side, would you wait until New Year's Day? Or until your birthday? Or until you went on holiday? Or would you make your move there and then?

Trying to plan the best time to make the change is a waste of time. There is only one correct answer:

DO IT NOW!

You have everything you need. Like an athlete on the blocks at the start of the 100 meters final, you are in the best position to fulfill one of the greatest achievements of your life RIGHT NOW!

Think of everything you have to gain. A life free from slavery, frustration, disappointment, anxiety, helplessness, and self-loathing. No more excuses, no more worrying about your health, no more missing out on genuine pleasures, and no more feeling powerless. Those dark days are gone as soon as you decide to make your move.

In their place, you can look forward to being in control of how you spend your time and money, enjoying exercise again as nature intended and rediscovering other genuine pleasures that you enjoyed before you became averse to exercise.

With so much happiness to gain and so much misery to shed, what possible reason is there to wait?

EIGHTH INSTRUCTION: DON'T WAIT FOR THE RIGHT TIME TO CHANGE, DO IT NOW!

Chapter 17

ENJOY LIFE

Now that you are near the end of the book, how do you feel? If you have followed all the instructions and understood everything I've explained, you should be brimming with excitement.

You picked up this book because you had a problem with exercise. Your motive in turning to Easyway was presumably to solve that problem. By choosing a method that works, you have achieved that and so much more.

You have opened your mind and identified the illusions that were responsible for keeping you trapped in lethargy. By following Easyway, you have removed those illusions. As a result, you will start enjoying regular exercise, a healthier diet, better sleep, greater physical fitness, greater mental peace, and a heightened zest for life. You are fully prepared.

You may still feel slightly apprehensive and unsure whether your new mindset will last. That's perfectly natural. What you are achieving is a major transformation, and you are bound to feel like you are in unfamiliar territory. Never doubt your decision to follow through on your commitment to exercise. With other major decisions we make, such as whom we marry or which job we choose, we can never know if they were correct. We may be perfectly happy with them, but we can never know what might have happened if we had done something else. The beauty of this decision is that you can be 100 percent certain that it is the correct decision even as you make it. So, having made what you know to be the right decision, never even begin to question or doubt it.

Trust in everything you have learned and very soon you will feel completely at ease with your new lifestyle. Remember, there is no need to wait for anything to happen before you start enjoying your new-found freedom. When you get into the groove of the virtuous circle of the right mindset, exercise, diet, and rest, it will gather its own unstoppable momentum.

LOOK AFTER YOURSELF

Your body is an incredible machine, capable of performing a multitude of tasks at the same time. Rejoice in the fact that you have this living, breathing machine and take pride in looking after it. Do that and the on-board computer will take care of everything else. It will tell you when the machine is fired up and raring to go and it will tell you when the machine needs to rest. As long as you respond to the signals, it will reward you with natural hormones that create happiness, positivity, and the motivation to repeat the cycle.

Eat well, exercise regularly, and respond when you feel pain or discomfort. Treat yourself kindly. After all, this is not just any machine we are talking about—this is YOU!

When you hear the words "health and fitness" you might picture an athlete, a personal trainer, or one of those people who likes to go out running for miles in the pouring rain, and you might be thinking, "That's just not me." No problem. Remember, exercise comes in many forms and is a pleasure in itself. Find a form or preferably several forms of exercise that you enjoy, a level that you are happy with and can sustain, and make it a natural, regular part of your life. It will very soon become second nature.

Of course, you are not going to be able to exercise as hard at the age of 80 as you did when you were 20—no one is asking you to. Your body will remain in balance as long as you pay attention to your fuel gauge and take in the fuel you need to match the energy you burn. How will you know? Because your body will tell you.

LEAD A BALANCED LIFE

When you get everything in balance—intake and output, activity and sleep, work and play—life feels easy. It's like having a perfectly tuned car. You don't think about what is going on under the hood; you just enjoy driving it. Your mind is free to think about positive, creative things. Things that make you happy.

It becomes self-perpetuating. The virtuous circle feeds on itself.

Remember the elements of that virtuous circle, and check up on them occasionally to ensure you are keeping everything in balance. It doesn't require much thought. You certainly don't need to stress about it. Just remember the importance of mindset, exercise, sleep, and diet in keeping that cycle going, and bear in mind that if any one of those elements becomes deficient, then the others will be affected.

Also, be careful not to overlook the balance between work and play. Some workaholics want to get fitter and sleep better just so they can go on flogging themselves to death with work. They want extra energy so they can work longer hours.

Remember, life should be fun. Working yourself into the ground impacts sleep, diet, and exercise, as well as tiring you out mentally. These factors in turn will negatively impact the quality of your work. Your energy, creative thinking, concentration, powers of organization, problem-solving ability, and other powers you need for work will diminish at an increasing rate. You will slow down, make mistakes, upset people, and get upset yourself. So, if you recognize these symptoms, check your balance. Chances are you are working worse, not better, and the rest of your life will suffer.

In order to have all your faculties functioning at full capacity, you need to balance work with rest and exercise. Getting all the rest you need doesn't mean you are lazy or work-shy. On the contrary, it shows that you take the trouble to maintain the incredible machine so it can operate at its optimal level. And the better the machine operates, the easier everything becomes.

THE PURSUIT OF HAPPINESS

Most people come to Easyway because they are not happy with at least one aspect of their life. For one reason or another, they are not living the life they want to live. Unhappiness is a clear signal from the incredible machine that something is wrong. It is a signal we are supposed to respond to, just as you would respond if a doctor told you that you had a life-threatening illness and needed to change some aspects of your lifestyle in order to avoid disaster. You have responded by picking up this book and reading it through to the end.

If you *have not* read the book all the way through to this point—if you have just skipped to the end, hoping to find a magic formula to solve your exercise problem—I'm very sorry, but it does not work that way.

Easyway is not magic. It is a very carefully constructed method based on first-hand experience and a deep understanding of the psychological struggles that affect us all. The method needs to be followed from start to finish. Miss out any part and it's like leaving out one digit from the combination to a safe. The door will remain locked.

If you *have* read the whole book to this point, congratulations! You have the complete combination to unlock the door. All you need to do now is use it.

NINTH INSTRUCTION: OPEN THE PRISON DOOR AND START ENJOYING LIFE TO THE FULLEST!

If you haven't done any exercise for a while, don't suddenly launch yourself into vigorous workouts right from the start, as that can cause injury and defeat your purpose. Ease yourself into it gradually and listen to any messages your body sends you. If you are at all concerned about this, you can always seek advice on the most appropriate level of exercise for you in your current condition and increase it as you become stronger. But don't feel that you have to conform to any regime imposed on you by anyone else because that's the way of willpower. You have taken back control. You don't want to relinquish it to someone else. Think about the moment when a dog is let out for its walk, or schoolchildren are let out into the playground. That burst of exuberance is what you should feel when the time comes to exercise. "This is fun!" "This is what I've been looking forward to!" "This is me time!"

Any doubts you had about having the necessary willpower or being capable of solving your exercise problem are now in the past. Any fears that changing your lifestyle would be hard and miserable are now far from your mind as you grow accustomed to the new exercise-friendly life you are living and all its benefits.

There is no reason to feel daunted. You are not being asked to climb Everest! You are still the same person you were when you first picked up this book. You are living almost the same life with a few adjustments that make a huge difference. You have not had to make any sacrifices. All that has gone from your life is the fog of illusions that had conned you into feeling stressed, anxious, and confused, and ultimately incapable of committing to exercise.

Those illusions were built up over your lifetime. It took just the time to absorb this book to remove them.

STAY STRONG

There will be times when you can't exercise or you find it harder than usual. I'm not pretending that your life will now be permanent bliss. That isn't real life, and there are always ups and downs. But now your baseline well-being will be higher than before, so the highs will be higher and the lows not as low. And if things do get tough, you will be stronger both physically and mentally and better able to handle any situation.

There will be worries, there will be stresses and strains, there will be times when you drink or take other drugs too much, or you spend too much time on social media, or you eat too much junk, or you don't get enough sleep. But now you don't need to panic. You understand the situation and you know what to do. It doesn't mean that everything you have learned and the changes you have made are wasted. You are not going to get fooled by those illusions again and you know how you will get back on track.

So when things seem to be against you, remain calm, pay attention to what your body is telling you, and check your balance. You know what you are looking for now and you know how to look. Make sure you are giving yourself the best chance of a good night's sleep. Check your diet for an excess of junk and ensure you are getting plenty of lovely fresh fruits and vegetables. Make sure the exercise you do is still a pleasure and if it isn't, change it to something else that you do enjoy.

By giving yourself these foundations, you will be better equipped to deal with whatever it is that is making life hard. The problem will pass, you will be stronger for it and better able to enjoy the highs of life to the full.

Chapter 18

FREEDOM

IN THIS CHAPTER

•*MORE HELP AND FREE-OF-CHARGE SUPPORT*

From time to time, it may help to have a quick reminder of the method and what you have learned along the way, so keep this book somewhere handy. For easy reference, here is a reminder of the instructions. It's good to take a look at them every now and then.

We have shown their associated chapters in case you want to reread any part.

1. Follow all the instructions. (Ch. 1)

2. Open your mind. (Ch. 2)

3. Begin with a feeling of excitement. (Ch. 4)

4. Ignore any advice that goes against Nature's guide. (Ch. 7)

5. Question your present tastes and eating habits. (Ch. 8)

6. Never doubt your decision to change. (Ch. 9)

7. Exercise for pleasure. (Ch. 14)

8. Don't wait for the right time to change, do it now! (Ch. 18)

9. Open the prison door and start enjoying life to the fullest! (Ch. 17)

You've done an amazing, wonderful thing. Once you feel in control of your exercise, truly enjoy it, and have incorporated it seamlessly into your everyday routine, there is no limit to what you can achieve in other areas of your life.

Congratulations on finishing the book and setting yourself free.

In the Appendix, there is a list of books and on-line video programs that might be of interest to you if you want to tackle any other addictive or behavioral issues, such as stopping smoking, losing weight or stopping drinking.

APPENDIX

MORE HELP AND FREE-OF-CHARGE SUPPORT

This book is a complete program in itself and I don't expect you to encounter any problems or issues at all, but please, if you feel the need to reach out for help, guidance, or advice, then do contact us via www.allencarr.com. We're always happy to hear from book readers—even if they need just a little extra advice, which is always provided free of charge. There is also a great Facebook group for people wanting to enjoy exercise—so feel free to check that out too. Search on Facebook for "Allen Carr's EASYWAY TO ENJOY EXERCISE" group.

The following list of books and on-line video programs might be of interest to you if you want to tackle any other addictive or behavioral issues in more detail.

Allen Carr's Easy Way to Quit Smoking Without Willpower: The latest upgrade of my stop-smoking method for life in the

2020s and beyond. It is also effective for those who use vapes, nicotine gum, Snus, or chewing tobacco/dip. This book will help you get free easily and painlessly.

Allen Carr's Easy Way to Quit Vaping: The latest upgrade of the method applied to vaping, heat-not-burn, or any other nicotine delivery system. Whether you used those products to quit smoking and now want to be free from all nicotine, or you've never smoked but got hooked on nicotine, this book will help you quit easily.

Allen Carr's Good Sugar, Bad Sugar: If you are overweight and your favorite foods are pizza, pasta, bread, potatoes, cakes, pastries, and candy, then it is likely that you have a sugar and carb issue. This is the latest upgrade of the method for getting free from ultra-processed foods and refined sugar.

Allen Carr's Easy Way to Quit Emotional Drinking: This is the latest upgrade of the method relating to alcohol, particularly if you feel your consumption is dictated by your emotions: stress, worry, and anxiety. This book will help you get free from the shackles of alcohol with ease.

Allen Carr's Easy Way to Quit Emotional Eating: Is your eating dictated to you by your emotions? Does stress, upset, worry, or anxiety fuel your consumption? This is the latest upgrade of the method relating to eating and will ensure with ease that your intake of food is prompted only by genuine hunger.

Allen Carr's Easy Way to Quit Cannabis: Have you wanted to cut down or quit cannabis in the past but failed to do so? It's likely that the feeling of sacrifice or of missing out on something you enjoy has prevented you from doing so. This book will enable you to get free without feeling any sense of loss.

Allen Carr's Easy Way to Quit Cocaine: Has cocaine started to eat away at your life—not just your money, your close relationships, friends, and job, but your sense of self-esteem, of self-worth, of who you really are? This book will set you free without any feelings of sacrifice.

Allen Carr's Easy Way to Better Sleep: Whether you've always had issues with getting enough sleep or it's something that's blighted you recently, this book will help you adopt tried and tested techniques to get free from insomnia. Even if you don't think you have a sleep problem but wake up most mornings feeling tired, this book is for you. It doesn't just focus on getting sleep, it focuses on getting GREAT sleep. Rather than implementing changes reluctantly, you'll be able to do so happily and easily.

Allen Carr's Easy Way to Mindfulness: If you've never explored mindfulness before or found it hard to practice, this book adapts the method to relieving everyday stress, anxiety, and depression through basic mindfulness techniques.

Allen Carr's Smart Phone, Dumb Phone: If you find it impossible to tear yourself from your phone, social media, messenger groups, tech, and gaming, this book will help you change your use from excessive levels to appropriate levels. You don't have to ditch your smart phone; you just have to enjoy its immense benefits without the downsides of overuse.

Allen Carr's Easy Way to Quit Caffeine: Do you always feel so tired that contemplating skipping coffee seems impossible? Do you feel that you are drinking far too much coffee far too often? This book will set you free from the control coffee and caffeine-laden energy drinks seem to have over you, eradicating your constant fatigue without feeling that you're missing out.

Allen Carr's Get Out of Debt Now: Stress, anxiety, and worry can be debilitating. When they are fueled by debt, they can be truly crippling—and worse. This book adapts the method to the task of becoming debt-free easily.

Allen Carr's Easy Way to Quit Gambling: Whether it's sports betting, on-line bingo, scratch cards, or full-on casino betting, this book will enable you to escape the ravages of compulsive gambling without feeling that you are sacrificing anything at all.

ALLEN CARR'S EASYWAY CENTERS

The following list indicates the countries where Allen Carr's Easyway To Stop Smoking Centers are currently operational.

Check www.allencarr.com for the latest additions to this list.

The success rate at the centers, based on the three-month, money-back guarantee, is over 90 percent.

Selected centers also offer sessions that deal with alcohol, other drugs, and sugar addiction/weight issues. Please check with your nearest center, listed on the following pages, for details.

Allen Carr's Easyway guarantees that you will find it easy to quit smoking, alcohol, or other drugs at our centers or your money back.

JOIN US!

Allen Carr's Easyway Centers have spread throughout the world with incredible speed and success. Our global franchise network now covers more than 150 cities in over 50 countries. This amazing growth has been achieved entirely organically. Former addicts, just like you, were so impressed by the ease with which they stopped that they felt inspired to contact us to see how they could bring the method to their region.

If you feel the same, contact us for details on how to become an Allen Carr's Easyway To Stop Smoking, an Allen Carr's Easyway To Stop Drinking, or an Allen Carr's Easyway to Quit Sugar franchisee.

Email us at join-us@allencarr.com, including your full name, postal address, and region of interest.

SUPPORT US!

No, don't send us money!

You have achieved something really marvelous. Every time we hear of someone escaping from the sinking ship, we get a feeling of enormous satisfaction.

It would give us great pleasure to hear that you have freed yourself from the slavery of addiction, so please visit the following web page where you can tell us of your success, inspire others to follow in your footsteps and hear about ways you can help to spread the word.

 www.allencarr.com/fanzone

 You can 'like' our Facebook page here:
www.facebook.com/AllenCarr

Together, we can help further Allen Carr's mission: to cure the world of addiction.

CENTERS

LONDON CENTER AND WORLDWIDE HEAD OFFICE
Park House, 14 Pepys Road,
Raynes Park, London SW20 8NH
Tel: +44 (0)20 8944 7761
Email: mail@allencarr.com
Website: www.allencarr.com
Therapists: John Dicey, Colleen
Dwyer, Crispin Hay, Emma Hudson,
Rob Fielding, Sam Kelser,
Rob Groves, Debbie Brewer-West,
Mark Keen, Duncan Bhaskaran-Brown,
Mark Newman, Gerry Williams
(alcohol) Monique Douglas (weight)

Worldwide Press Office
Contact: John Dicey
Tel: +44 (0)7970 88 44 52
Email: media@allencarr.com

NORTH AMERICA

USA
Sessions held throughout the USA
Tel: +1 855 440 3777
Email: support@usa.allencarr.com
Website: www.allencarr.com

Los Angeles
Tel: +1 855 440 3777
Therapists: Natalie Clays and team
Email: support@usa.allencarr.com
Website: www.allencarr.com

Milwaukee (and South Wisconsin)
Tel: +1 262 770 1260
Therapist: Wayne Spaulding
Email: wayne@easywaywisconsin.com
Website: www.allencarr.com

New York
Tel: +1 855 440 3777
Therapists: Natalie Clays and team
Email: support@usa.allencarr.com
Website: www.allencarr.com

CANADA
Tel: +1 (0)855 440 3777
Therapist: Natalie Clays
Email: natalie@ca.allencarr.com
Website: www.allencarr.com

UK CENTERS

UK Center Information and Central Booking Line
Tel: 0800 389 2115 (UK only)

Birmingham

Bournemouth

Brentwood

Brighton

Bristol

Cambridge

Cumbria

Derby

Kent

Lancashire

Liverpool

Milton Keynes

Newcastle/North East

Nottingham

Oxford

Reading

Southampton

Southport

Staines/Heathrow

Stevenage

Stoke

Watford
Tel: 0800 389 2115
Therapists: John Dicey, Colleen Dwyer, Crispin Hay, Emma Hudson, Rob Fielding, Sam Kelser, Rob Groves, Debbie Brewer-West, Mark Keen, Duncan Bhaskaran-Brown, Mark Newman
Email: mail@allencarr.com
Website: www.allencarr.com

Coventry
Tel: 0800 321 3007
Therapist: Rob Fielding
Email: info@easywaymidlands.co.uk
Website: www.allencarr.com

Isle of Man
Tel: 0800 077 6187
Therapist: Mark Keen
Email: mark@easywaymanchester.co.uk
Website: www.allencarr.com

Leeds
Tel: 0800 077 6187
Therapist: Mark Keen
Email: mark@easywaymanchester.co.uk
Website: www.allencarr.com

Leicester
Tel: 0800 321 3007
Therapist: Rob Fielding
Email: info@easywaymidlands.co.uk
Website: www.allencarr.com

Lincoln
Tel: 0800 321 3007
Therapist: Rob Fielding
Email: info@easywaymidlands.co.uk
Website: www.allencarr.com

Manchester
Tel: 0800 077 6187
Therapist: Mark Keen
Email: mark@easywaymanchester.co.uk
Website: www.allencarr.com

Surrey
Park House, 14 Pepys Road, Raynes
Park, London SW20 8NH
Tel: +44 (0)20 8944 7761
Fax: +44 (0)20 8944 8619
Therapists: John Dicey, Colleen
Dwyer, Crispin Hay, Emma Hudson,
Rob Fielding, Sam Kelser, Rob
Groves, Debbie Brewer-West,
Mark Keen, Duncan Bhaskaran-
Brown, Mark Newman, Gerry
Williams (Alcohol) Monique
Douglas (Weight)
Email: mail@allencarr.com
Website: www.allencarr.com

Worcester
Tel: 0800 321 3007
Therapist: Rob Fielding
Email: info@easywaymidlands.co.uk
Website: www.allencarr.com

GUERNSEY
Tel: 0800 077 6187
Therapist: Mark Keen
Email: mark@easywaymanchester.co.uk
Website: www.allencarr.com

JERSEY
Tel: 0800 077 6187
Therapist: Mark Keen
Email: mark@easywaymanchester.co.uk
Website: www.allencarr.com

SCOTLAND
Glasgow and Edinburgh
Tel: +44 (0)131 449 7858
Therapists: Paul Melvin and Jim
McCreadie
Email: info@easywayscotland.co.uk
Website: www.allencarr.com

WORLDWIDE CENTERS

AUSTRALIA

ACT, NSW, NT, QLD, VIC
Tel: 1300 848 028
Therapist: Natalie Clays and Team
Email: natalie@allencarr.com.au
Website: www.allencarr.com

South Australia

Tel: 1300 848 028
Therapist: Jaime Reed
Email: sa@allencarr.com.au
Website: www.allencarr.com

Western Australia

Tel: 1300 848 028
Therapist: Natalie Clays and Team
Email: natalie@allencarr.com.au
Website: www.allencarr.com

AUSTRIA

Sessions held throughout Austria
Freephone: 0800RAUCHEN
(0800 7282436)
Tel: +43 (0)3512 44755
Therapists: Erich Kellermann
and Team
Email: info@allen-carr.at
Website: www.allencarr.com

BELGIUM

Brussels
Tel: +32 (02) 808 19 65
Therapist: Paula Rooduijn
Email: info@allencarr.be
Website: www.allencarr.com

BRAZIL

Therapist: Lilian Brunstein
Email: contato@easywayonline.com.br
Website: www.allencarr.com

BULGARIA

Tel: 0800 14104/+359 899 88 99 07
Therapist: Rumyana Kostadinova
Email: rk@nepushaveche.com
Website: www.allencarr.com

CHILE

Tel: +56 2 4744587
Therapist: Claudia Sarmiento
Email: contacto@allencarr.cl
Website: www.allencarr.com

CYPRUS

Tel: +357 25770611
Therapist: Andreas Damianou
Email: info@allencarr.com.cy
Website: www.allencarr.com

DENMARK

Sessions held throughout Denmark
Tel: +45 70267711
Therapist: Mette Frnss
Email: mette@easyway.dk
Website: www.allencarr.com

ESTONIA
Tel: +372 733 0044
Therapist: Henry Jakobson
Email: info@allencarr.ee
Website: www.allencarr.com

FINLAND
Tel: +358-(0)45 3544099
Therapist: Janne Ström
Email: info@allencarr.fi
Website: www.allencarr.com

FRANCE
Sessions held throughout France
Freephone: 0800 386387
Tel: +33 (4) 91 33 54 55
Therapists: Erick Serre and Team
Email: info@allencarr.fr
Website: www.allencarr.com

GERMANY
Sessions held throughout Germany
Freephone: 08000RAUCHEN
(0800 07282436)
Tel: +49 (0) 8031 90190-0
Therapists: Erich Kellermann
and Team
Email: info@allen-carr.de
Website: www.allencarr.com

GREECE
Sessions held throughout Greece
Tel: +30 210 5224087
Therapist: Panos Tzouras
Email: panos@allencarr.gr
Website: www.allencarr.com

GUATEMALA
Tel: +502 2362 0000
Therapist: Michelle Binford
Email: info@dejadefumarfacil.com
Website: www.allencarr.com

HONG KONG
Email: info@easywayhongkong.com
Website: www.allencarr.com

HUNGARY
Seminars in Budapest and 12 other
cities across Hungary
Tel: 06 80 624 426 (freephone) or
+36 20 580 9244
Therapist: Gábor Szász
email: szasz.gabor@allencarr.hu
Website: www.allencarr.com

INDIA
Bangalore & Chennai
Tel: +91 (0)80 4154-0624
Therapist: Suresh Shottam
Email: info@easywaytostopsmoking.
co.in
Website: www.allencarr.com

IRAN
Please check website for details
Tehran and Mashhad
Website: www.allencarr.com

ISRAEL
Sessions held throughout Israel
Tel: +972 (0)3 6212525
Therapists: Orit Rozen and team
Email: info@allencarr.co.il
Website: www.allencarr.com

ITALY
Sessions held throughout Italy
Tel: +39 (0)2 7060 2438
Therapists: Francesca Cesati
and team
Email: info@easywayitalia.com
Website: www.allencarr.com

JAPAN
Sessions held throughout Japan
www.allencarr.com

LEBANON
Tel: +961 1 791 5565
Therapist: Sadek El-Assaad
Email: info@AllenCarrEasyWay.me
Website: www.allencarr.com

MAURITIUS
Tel: +230 5727 5103
Therapist: Heidi Hoareau
Email: info@allencarr.mu
Website: www.allencarr.com

MEXICO
Sessions held throughout Mexico
Tel: +52 55 2623 0631
Therapist: Jorge Davo and team
Email: info@allencarr-mexico.com
Website: www.allencarr.com

NETHERLANDS
Sessions held throughout the
Netherlands
Allen Carr's Easyway 'stoppen met
roken'
Tel: +31 53 478 43 62/
+31 900 786 77 37
Email: info@allencarr.nl
Website: www.allencarr.com

NEW ZEALAND
North Island – Auckland
Tel: +64 (0) 0800 848 028
Therapist: Natalie Clays and team
Email: natalie@allencarr.co.nz
Website: www.allencarr.com

South Island – Wellington and Christchurch
Tel: +64 (0) 0800 848 028
Therapist: Natalie Clays and Team
Email: natalie@allencarr.co.nz

NORWAY
Therapist: Laila Thorsen
Please check website for details
Website: www.allencarr.com

PERU – Lima
Tel: +511 637 7310
Therapist: Luis Loranca
Email: lloranca@
dejardefumaraltoque.com
Website: www.allencarr.com

POLAND
Sessions throughout Poland
Tel: +48 (0) 22 621 36 11
Therapist: Michael Spyrka
Email: info@allen-carr.pl
Website: www.allencarr.com

POLAND – Alcohol sessions
Tel: +48 71 307 32 37
Therapist: Maciej Kramarz
Email: mk@allecarr.com.pl
Website: www.allencarr.com

PORTUGAL
Oporto
Tel: +351 22 9958698
Therapist: Ria Slof
Email: info@comodeixardefumar.com
Website: www.allencarr.com

REPUBLIC OF IRELAND
Dublin
Tel: +353 (0)1 499 9010
Therapists: Paul Melvin & Jim McCreadie
Email: info@allencarr.ie
Website: www.allencarr.com

ROMANIA
Tel: +40 (0) 7321 3 8383
Therapist: Cristina Nichita
Email: raspunsuri@allencarr.ro
Website: www.allencarr.com

RUSSIA
Allen Carr's Easyway to Stop Smoking
Live Seminars & Online Video Program
Tel: +7 495 644 64 26
Freecall +7 (800) 250 6622
Therapist: Alexander Fomin
Email: info@allencarr.ru
Website: www.allencarr.com

RUSSIA
Allen Carr's Easyway to Stop Drinking
Live Seminars & Online Video Program
Tel: +8 (800) 302 80 68/
+7 985 207 47 93
Therapist: Artem Kasyanov
Email: info@allencarrlife.ru
Website: www.allencarr.com

St Petersburg
Please check website for details
Website: www.allencarr.com

SERBIA
Belgrade
Tel: +381 (0)11 308 8686
Email: office@allencarr.co.rs
Website: www.allencarr.com

SINGAPORE
Tel: +65 62241450
Therapist: Pam Oei
Email: pam@allencarr.com.sg
Website: www.allencarr.com

SLOVENIA
Tel: +386 (0) 40 77 61 77
Therapist: Grega Sever
Email: easyway@easyway.si
Website: www.allencarr.com

SOUTH AFRICA
Sessions held throughout South
Africa
National Booking Line: 0861 100 200
Head Office: 15 Draper Square,
Draper St, Claremont 7708,
Cape Town
Cape Town: Dr Charles Nel
Tel: +27 (0)21 851 5883
Mobile: 083 600 5555
Therapists: Dr Charles Nel, Malcolm
Robinson and team
Email: easyway@allencarr.co.za
Website: www.allencarr.com

SOUTH KOREA – SEOUL
Tel: +82 (0)70 4227 1862
Therapist: Yousung Cha
Email: master@allencarr.co.kr
Website: www.allencarr.com

SPAIN
Tel: +34 910 05 29 99
Therapist: Luis Loranca
Email: informes@AllenCarrOfficial.es
Website: www.allencarr.com

SWEDEN
Tel: +46 70 695 6850
Therapists: Nina Ljungqvist, Renée
Johansson
Email: info@easyway.se
Website: www.allencarr.com

SWITZERLAND
Sessions held throughout
Switzerland
Freephone: 0800RAUCHEN
(0800 / 728 2436)
Tel: +41 (0)52 383 3773
Therapists: Cyrill Argast and team
For sessions in Suisse Romand and
Svizzera Italiana
Tel: 0800 386 387
Email: info@allen-carr.ch
Website: www.allencarr.com

TURKEY
Sessions held throughout Turkey
Tel: +90 212 358 5307
Therapist: Emre Üstünuçar
Email: info@allencarr.com.tr
Website: www.allencarr.com

UNITED ARAB EMIRATES
Dubai and Abu Dhabi
Tel: +97 56 693 4000
Therapist: Sadek El-Assaad
Email: info@AllenCarrEasyWay.me
Website: www.allencarr.com

Easyway publications are also available as audiobooks.

Visit shop.allencarr.com to find out more.

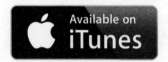 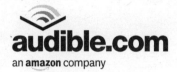